What Is Life and How Might It Be Sustained?

How did the universe and life begin and what are the threats to people and the environment in a pandemic? This book is for anybody with an interest in protecting life on the planet. Studies on the origin of life and scientific contributions to safeguarding the planet are examined in light of current thinking on climate change. A major focus is the spread of microbes, put in the context of environmental assessment and management, including descriptions of microbiomes and a consideration of the risks of genetic modifications. Prof. Lynch shows how failure to control disease can lead to the collapse of any biotic population. To avoid this, the ethics of management of disease by biological control and by vaccination are discussed, at the practical level and in a moral theological context.

What Is Life and How Might It Be Sustained?

Reflections in a Pandemic

Jim Lynch

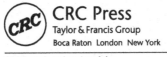

CRC Press
Taylor & Francis Group
Boca Raton London New York

CRC Press is an imprint of the
Taylor & Francis Group, an **Informa** business

Cover image description: The Power of Imaging at Micro and Global Levels
The front cover depicts a microbiome of various bacteria within the human gut and uses the power of scanning electron microscopic imaging (Getty Images). The rear cover shows fishbone and mosaic deforestation in the Amazon rainforest at Rondonia in Brazil with the power of DMC-2 satellite imagery at 22 m resolution, incorporating an amplified insert; the forest area is red, and the logged area is blue (Airbus).

First edition published 2023
by CRC Press
6000 Broken Sound Parkway NW, Suite 300, Boca Raton, FL 33487-2742

and by CRC Press
4 Park Square, Milton Park, Abingdon, Oxon, OX14 4RN

CRC Press is an imprint of Taylor & Francis Group, LLC

Library of Congress Cataloging-in-Publication Data
Names: Lynch, J. M. (James Michael) author.
Title: What is life and how might it be sustained? : reflections in a pandemic / Jim Lynch.
Description: Fourth edition. | Boca Raton : CRC Press, 2023. |
Includes bibliographical references and index. |
Identifiers: LCCN 2022007757 (print) | LCCN 2022007758 (ebook) |
ISBN 9781032303888 (hardback) | ISBN 9781032275475 (paperback) |
ISBN 9781003304845 (ebook)
Subjects: LCSH: Life—Origin. | Environmental protection. |
Communicable diseases—Prevention. | Extinction (Biology)
Classification: LCC QH325 .L96 2023 (print) | LCC QH325 (ebook) |
DDC 576.8/3—dc23/eng/20220411
LC record available at https://lccn.loc.gov/2022007757
LC ebook record available at https://lccn.loc.gov/2022007758

ISBN: 978-1-032-30388-8 (hbk)
ISBN: 978-1-032-27547-5 (pbk)
ISBN: 978-1-003-30484-5 (ebk)

DOI: 10.1201/9781003304845

Typeset in Times
by codeMantra

Access the eResource: https://www.routledge.com/9781032303888

To MARY

My wife, who has not only improved so many of my manuscripts over 50 years of our marriage, but also gave me four such great children, Luke, Dominic, Cordelia, and Francesca, who in turn with their spouses have given us seven such wonderful grandchildren, Nathaniel, Tobias, Finnian, Alannah, Rufus, Tallulah, and Imogen. Tallulah was born May 2021 in Washington, DC where the Cosmology chapter was written, and Imogen was born June 2021 in London where the Origins of Life chapter was written.

Contents

Foreword

With grace and candour, Jim Lynch provides sensitive and thoughtful discourse on the most meaningful of questions. The origin of life and the nature of goodness and evil are amongst the many topics probed in this book and each is crafted in keen scientific thought. The issues are presented in a cosmic framework: food security, human health, deforestation, climate change, and pandemics. COVID-19, the contemporary global pandemic afflicting all nations, is addressed scientifically but also as a philosophical and ethical challenge. Jim Lynch brings to each of these issues a solid background in chemistry, biochemistry, microbiology, soil science, agricultural science, philosophy, and ethics.

The intertwining of religion and science is achieved both deliberatively and intellectually by thoughtful weighing of the issues yet piercing through to rational conclusions.

Most intriguing are his life experiences as one who has mastered academic challenges and walked a path of scientific research, science policy, and policy making. His background in soil microbiology, agricultural production, and health policy provides a foundation of knowing the walk – not just the talk. Having been involved in many facets of agricultural production – improving crops genetically and fighting diseases of agriculturally important crops, e.g., wheat but also of domestic animals – his advice on food parity for lesser developed countries and for actions to curb climate change rings true.

In this book, Jim Lynch has penned thoughts and reflections, sharing both wisdom and advice, at a time of planetary crisis, when we are all in a seemingly never-ending pandemic, worsening climate change, fractious leaders of key nation states threatening violence, and public decline in civility. Yet hope prevails and the message from these thoughtful and candid musings is reassuring – science and religion are not mutually exclusive but interactive, with both necessary to explain life and how it can be sustained. Jim's optimism, fortunately, is infectious.

Rita R. Colwell

Preface

When the COVID-19 virus was first identified in Wuhan, China, in November 2019, few people realised the pandemic that would emerge. Especially with quarantine measures, it gave everybody a chance to think about life and death. I had researched the origin of bacterial life during my PhD studies, and the pandemic presented an opportunity to consider the meaning of life in all its forms and how it might be protected. I started to discuss my ideas with Alice Oven at CRC Press within the Taylor & Francis Group in early February 2021 and agreed to produce this book by the end of that year. The period of the pandemic was a challenging time for science but against most expectations vaccines against the virus were developed quickly. By the time I submitted the manuscript on the due date, the vaccination programme was reducing the viral threat, especially in developed countries. Even the emergence of a new Omicron variant fortunately did not seem to be such a threat to life as the previously dominant Delta variant. However, it would be misplaced complacency to think that the threat had disappeared as the virus moves to an endemic phase. For example, with endemic malaria, more than 600,000 people died in 2020. The story of dying in the twenty-first century is something of a paradox, as indicated in the *Lancet* Commission on the Value of Death: bringing death back into life, published in January 2022. Many people are overtreated, still more remain undertreated, dying from preventable conditions and without access to basic pain relief. People died during pandemic often alone and unable to communicate with family. Death and life are bound together; without death, there would be no life, and this has been explored for centuries by philosophers and theologians. Caring for the dying is a gift, especially with the recent achievements of the hospice movement, and to rebalance death, dying and grieving, radical changes across all death systems are needed. For example, realistic change has been achieved in Kerala, India, over three decades by social movement with tens of thousands of volunteers.

The COVID-19 pandemic has often led to the recognition that it is a delusion that we are in control and not part of nature. A similar situation exists with the problems of climate change which affect life. This book mentions COP26 which took place in November 2021 and even though agreement on emissions targets was limited, there was a pledge by 100 countries to reduce emissions of methane, which is 28 times as potent as carbon dioxide as a global warming gas, by 30% over the period of 2020–2030. However, an article published in *Nature* in February 2022 indicates that methane is now spiking. Microbes seem to be responsible for about 85% in growth in emissions since 2007, with the remainder being due to fossil fuel extraction. Wetlands are the primary culprit at 161.6 million tonnes per year, followed by fossil fuel extraction (129.5), livestock (103), and landfill and agricultural waste (72.9). This demonstrates that a holistic approach needs to be taken to manage life on our planet, and microbes are often at the heart of our problems but can also generate opportunities. My early research of methane-utilising bacteria indicated that they were probably pioneer species on earth although it would be optimistic to think they could be harnessed for the current problem of methane. However, the soil and plants, especially the regions around roots, are good targets for microbe management as covered in my earlier books on *Soil Biotechnology* (1983) and *The Rhizosphere* (1990), especially as regulators become more sensitive about exposure to potentially harmful chemicals.

Superficially, it might appear that maximising plant biomass on the planet would improve carbon capture and mitigate climate change. However, the planting of non-native Sitka spruce in the post-World War II period in the UK to generate maximum woody biomass generated problems in terms of soil erosion and loss of biodiversity. Similar problems have been reported at the start of 2022 in Wales with Sitka spruce as people chase the financial incentives of carbon credits. All actions that we take to manage our planet must be sustainable and this is where life cycle assessment is critical.

In January 2022, the Foundation for Science and Technology organised a discussion meeting on how the National Science and Technology Council, chaired by the Prime Minister, and the Office for Science and Technology led by Sir Patrick Vallance as Chief Scientific and National Technology Advisor, should direct its priorities. The four key areas are to be:

1. Sustainable environment
2. Health and life sciences
3. National security and defence, including space
4. A digitally and data-driven economy

This is good news, and to achieve this, it will be critical that industry and the financial institutions work with the public sector and universities to achieve the objectives. They reflect much of the ground that is covered in this book; even objective 3 is being harnessed by using earth observation with satellites to improve land use and monitor the achievement of the UN Sustainable Development Goals. Hopefully, the areas will be interactive. Medicine was traditionally called physic and there was a strong emphasis on the use of plants in medicine. There still seems to be great opportunity in objective 2 to harness the natural environment as we move forward to try to improve life on earth while recognising how much we already owe to the pharmaceutical industry. This book will hopefully support integrated thinking on life and show how harnessing modern science can give grounds for optimism for the future.

Acknowledgements

In attempting to interact with people in the various branches of mathematics, science, including social sciences, and religion, I have greatly enjoyed exploring the interfaces in writing this book. At Wilson's Grammar School, I was privileged to be taught by enthusiasts such as Geoff Barraclough who subsequently went on to teach chemistry in Africa, before coming back to the UK to become Chair of the Association of Science Education. I was also exposed to physical activity as a joy of life which I have continued throughout my life, especially athletics, by Philip Johnson who went on to become Head of Sports and Recreation at City University London. Running, cycling, kayaking, sailing, golf, and walking have been a great comfort to me at times of stress.

I am ever grateful to BP for scholarships that enabled me to study BTech industrial chemistry at Loughborough University and then PhD and DSc in Microbiology at Queen Elizabeth (now King's) College in London. At the Letcombe Laboratory and Oxford University where I taught soil biotechnology, I had a great team of colleagues such as Malcolm Drew and John Whipps, and research students such as Stephen Harper and Duncan Veal. While there and subsequently at Horticulture Research International where John Whipps joined me, I benefitted from working with many great research students, postdoctoral fellows, and collaborators such as Mark Bailey and Pat Harvey. I was also able to enjoy sabbaticals as Visiting Professor and at Washington State University and then Oregon State Universities funded as Distinguished Scientist by the United States Department of Agriculture with my great friend and colleague Lloyd Elliott. I also enjoyed greatly my periods as Visiting Professor at King's College London, working with the late Michael Bazin, John Pirt, and Clive Bird, at the University of Reading working with John Grainger, and the University of Helsinki, working with Heikki Hokkanen. It was also great to have visitors from abroad such as Bob Lumsden, Don Crawford, Doug Eveleigh, Bernard Glick, and Balu Chopade in my various laboratories on sabbaticals. Spending at least one quarter of my time abroad some years, I had so much pleasure at being able to stay with colleagues in their homes. When I moved to the University of Surrey in 1993, my colleague Frans De Leij came with me from HRI to run my research laboratory and I was able to benefit from interdisciplinary collaboration with people like Glynis Breakwell, Roland Clift, Steve Morse, Richard Murphy, Jhuma Sadhukhan Martin Sweeting, and Ian Roulstone as well as many outstanding research students and postdoctoral fellows, especially lately Mercio Cerbaro and Ana Andries. While at Surrey, I was also able benefit from collaboration with Rita Colwell at the University of Maryland, and she became the first biologist and was the first woman to become Director of the National Science Foundation in the United States. I am privileged that she has written the Foreword of this book. I was able to retain my association at Surrey during my four-year period at the Forestry Commission as CEO of the Research Agency and subsequently as Distinguished Professor of Life Sciences, which is now an emeritus role. I have also been privileged to benefit from the support of the Earl of Selborne until his death in 2021.

I was extremely lucky to have Alice Oven, Life Sciences Editor of Taylor & Francis Group/CRC Press, to support me throughout the writing and production of the book. She was ably assisted by Shikha Garg, while I was also supported on IT problems as they emerged by my sailing skipper Geoff Tricker. I thank them all.

I am very grateful to those who have read various parts of this book for me and engaged in stimulating discussion, including Stephen Morse, Johnjoe McFadden, John Whipps, Frans De Leij, Bob Lumsden, Canon David Parmiter, Bishop Richard Moth, Bishop Richard Cheetham, Xavier Calmet, Glynis Breakwell, Peter Williams, Dominic Whitehouse, and Michael Heathcote. My wife Mary has not only made comments on this book, but on so much of what I have written during my career, and I am so grateful to her for tolerating me in the highs and lows of an interdisciplinary career in science. Fortunately, it is the highs that I remember most, leaving me no regrets on my career path.

Author

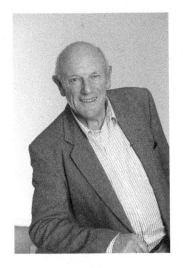

Jim Lynch graduated with BTech in Industrial Chemistry from Loughborough University, and then completed his PhD and DSc in Microbiology at Kings College London. He is a Fellow of the Royal Society of Chemistry, the Royal Society of Biology, the Royal Geographical Society, the Royal Society of Arts, and is a Chartered Chemist, Biologist, Scientist, and Environmentalist. He has worked at BBSRC research institutes, universities as visiting professor (Oxford, Reading, Kings College London, Imperial College, Washington State, Oregon State and Helsinki), and companies as non-executive director or advisor. Prof. Lynch was Dean of Biomedical and Life Sciences, University of Surrey, Chief Executive of the Forestry Commission Research Agency, Chairman of the Biology Division of the International Union of Soil Sciences, Coordinator of the OECD Research Programme on Biological Resource Management, Board Member of the European Forest Institute, Chair of Governors University of Chichester, and is Distinguished Professor of Life Sciences Emeritus at the Centre for Environment and Sustainability, University of Surrey. He has travelled extensively giving more than 60 keynote international lectures and published or edited 15 books previously and 300 papers and patents, as well as serving on many international boards. He was awarded the UNESCO Prize in Microbiology and Einstein Medal, Distinguished Scientist of the US Department of Agriculture, and the Japanese Government Research Award for Foreign Specialists. He is an Officer of the Order of the British Empire (*OBE*), a Knight of the Equestrian Order of the Holy Sepulchre of Jerusalem (*KHS*), and a Freeman of the City of London. Prof. Lynch is a keen sportsman and is married to Mary; they have four children and seven grandchildren.

1 Introduction

The most beautiful thing we can experience is the mysterious. It is the source of all true art and science. He to whom the emotion is a stranger, who can no longer pause to wonder, and stand wrapped in awe, is as good as dead – his eyes are closed. The insight into the mystery of life, coupled though it be with fear, has also given rise to religion. To know what is impenetrable to us really exists, manifesting itself as the highest wisdom and the most radiant beauty, which our dull faculties can comprehend only in their most primitive forms – this knowledge, this feeling is at the center of true religiousness.

Albert Einstein, 1879–1955

Look after the land and the land will look after you, destroy the land and it will destroy you.

Aboriginal proverb

If we lose the land, we lose the culture. Lose the culture, lose the peace. Lose the peace, lose the community. Lose the community, lose our way of life. Forever.

Oloiboni Kitok, Maasai spiritual leader.

This book will discuss how was life created, what are the threats to life as we know it, and how might it be managed sustainably to secure life on the planet. The coronavirus pandemic has changed the world as we know it. The scientific world has come together in an unprecedented way to attempt to combat the virus, and there is a new familiarity amongst many with the work of scientists, medical practitioners and epidemiologists, and sociologists. However, discipline boundaries can often seem impenetrable even though breaking them down is critical to our future. The virus has rendered us vulnerable in a way we never thought possible. We have come to realise that life is fragile, especially when our activities have led to global warming to threaten life. This exposure to uncertainty has led many to question what we value as global and local communities, and what is now compromised. Management of land is crucial in this. Some may ponder on the origin of life itself and the threats to its future existence. In the throes of the pandemic, there is a new consciousness of the need for a better world in which human communities and their associated biota can lead a healthy and sustainable life. The age-old conflict between science and religion continues, but is there a way they can work together for the benefit of mankind?

Quantum physics is a key factor in the origin of life. The term quantum physics has entered public consciousness via the work of Stephen Hawking and the television documentaries by Brian Cox. *The Grand Design* (2010) by Stephen Hawking and Leonard Mlodinow introduced the reading public to the subject. Roger Penrose, Stephen's PhD examiner, had described how quantum physics shapes the way we think in his book *Shadows of the Mind* (1995). Penrose received the 2020 Nobel Prize in Physics for his work on black hole formation, one of the most important

DOI: 10.1201/9781003304845-1

phenomena of the universe, as a predictor of the general theory of relativity. Stephen addressed the timeless questions of life on this planet in his book published just after his death *Brief Answers to Big Questions* (2018). My colleague Johnjoe McFadden introduced *Quantum Evolution* (2000) in which he describes this new science of life and how it may have emerged from the primeval soup. Johnjoe collaborated with another colleague, quantum physicist Jim Al-Khalili, and in their book *Life on the Edge* (2014) described how very small events in the quantum world can affect creatures such as us.

The great question remains where do we come from? What was the spark to create life? Physical events almost certainly initiate the pathway for a route to life, but the primary trigger is still unclear and remains a mystery. Such events must be followed by chemical organisation of molecules, and I had the opportunity to pursue this topic for my PhD while funded by the oil company BP who had also generously funded my undergraduate studies. Initially, I found that the lipid fraction of fungi is a source of long-chain hydrocarbons. Further research on a methane-utilising bacterium, *Methylococcus capsulatus* (Figure 1.1), being grown in bulk by Shell as a possible food source revealed that the dominant hydrocarbon, accounting for 0.5% of its cell mass, was squalene with a carbon chain length of 30 in a branched structure made up of six isoprene units. This appeared to be associated with the extensive internal membranes structure of the bacterium. At that time (1971), it was believed that the lowest class of cells, prokaryotes which are bacteria and blue-green algae,

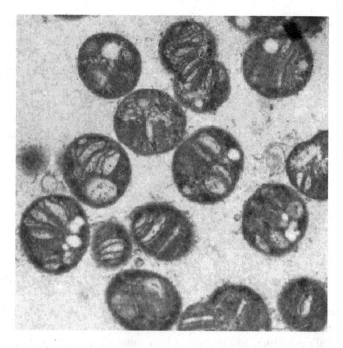

FIGURE 1.1 *Methylococcus capsulatus.* The cells are 1 micrometre in diameter and the cells have a dense internal membrane system containing squalene. (With permission from Anne Fjellbirkeland)

had the absence of sterols as a distinguishing chemical feature. Surely squalene in the methane-utilising bacterium could not be metabolised to sterols? Instrumental techniques were inadequate at the time, and although gas chromatography (GC) was an option to separate them, it would not identify the chemical structures. For identification, a mass spectrometer (MS) would need to be coupled to the flame ionisation detector of the GC. The problem was that hardly any such devices were available. At Bristol University, they had just received the samples of lunar rocks from the first Moon Landing and were using combined GC-MS to analyse them. A trip to Bristol was unsuccessful as the sterols which had been analysed by GC on glass columns in my laboratory in London stuck to the walls of the steel columns being used in Bristol. Another GC-MS system became available at Glasgow University which used glass columns and identified the presence of two unusual sterols. This was the first demonstration of sterols in prokaryotes, resulting in a revision of the distinction between eukaryotes and this was published in *Nature*. This was of great interest to BP because using the new technique with glass capillary columns and working with a group at Strasbourg University they had found some very ancient (2.7 billion years) sediments, the Soudan Shales in Minnesota, chemical structures which were the same as those in the bacterium. This research was therefore indicative that methane-utilising bacteria, which are capable of growth up to 50°C were probably the oldest forms of life on the planet, making use of methane in the primordial atmosphere. Such markers have never been found on the Moon, but they will likely be investigated when Martian samples come to earth. Methane is of great concern today in global warming because it has about 30 times the global warming potential of carbon dioxide. It is perhaps surprising that the methanotrophic bacteria that utilise methane have received little attention in relation to their potential to remove methane from the atmosphere.

Many ideas have been promulgated to describe how chemical reactions from a big spark in the primordial atmosphere may have led to life on the planet. These were catalogued by Nobel laureate Melvin Calvin in his book on *Chemical Evolution* (1961) and will be discussed in this volume, alongside more recent ideas by Gaia Vince in her book *Adventures in the Anthropocene* (2014) and by Michael Marshall in his book *The Genesis Quest* (2020). Of particular interest are the Miller Urey experiments in which a spark was generated in a synthesised atmosphere thought to be representative of the primordial atmosphere of the earth and detected biological molecules are present in living cells. Beyond the sparks, I will try to show primitive cells formed, leading to microorganisms which have beneficial impacts on us we evolved, but also discuss some of the harm they can cause.

In the mid-twentieth century, a controversial Jesuit priest, Pierre Teilhard de Chardin, who was a geologist and palaeontologist, excited considerable interest with his ideas on evolution and the origin of life. Palaeontology investigates fossil structures, building from the chemical evidence just described. Teilhard in his book *The Phenomenon of Man* (1955, English Translation 1959) outlined evolution as the transition from an abiotic to biotic state. He described a synthetic model of evolution linking to cosmic theology. The evolutionary biologist Sir Julian Huxley praised elements of his work, in contrast to the scornful review delivered by the immunologist and Nobel laureate Peter Medawar, and later by the ethologist and evolutionary biologist Richard Dawkins. Teilhard's views brought him into much conflict with the Catholic Church, just as Galileo Galilei had effectively been isolated by the Church for his views of the Earth and its place in the solar system. In more recent times, Teilhard's vision of the world has found support from esteemed quarters, notably Cardinal Ratzinger, subsequently Pope Benedict XVI. This volume will delve further into the legacy of Teilhard's work.

The twenty-first century has brought us a challenge unlike any other we have faced – saving life on earth. We have ignored warning signs which have been clear for at least six decades, and the clock is still ticking. Rachel Carson identified the threads in her book *Silent Spring* (1962). She described how pesticides threatened the delicate balance of nature, and how irresponsible crop-dusting has decimated countless forms of life. Indeed, human life itself may well be endangered by pesticides. Such a view generated hostility in the agrochemical industry, especially as she was a marine biologist. This was book strongly supported by Julian Huxley in writing the Preface and was influential in Jim Lovelock writing the book *Gaia. A New Look at Life on Earth* (1979). Lovelock had an outstanding reputation as a scientist, having developed the use of the flame ionisation detector in GC, and worked with NASA in their space programme. As an independent scientist and choosing to work from a cottage in the West of Ireland, he brought knowledge from astronomy to zoology in support of his hypothesis that the earth functions as a single organism which defines and maintains conditions necessary for its survival, developing a radically different model of earth. He had the support of many colleagues, especially Lynn Margulis of Boston University. One of the principal opponents of his hypothesis was Richard Dawkins of Oxford University who argued that there is no way for natural selection to lead to altruism global in scale. His concept of Mother Earth of Gaia as the Greeks called it long ago excited much debate and discussion which continues today. In 2015, Pope Francis, who was a chemical technician by training in Argentina before studying philosophy and theology, wrote a very important Encyclical letter *Laudato Si'. On Care for Our Common Home*. In the Encyclical, he put the case to protect the environment along the lines of the Gaia hypothesis. Significant individuals who have championed the cause have included David Attenborough with his outstanding television programmes, which include warning of the dangers to wildlife of plastics in the environment. Also, HRH Prince Charles with Tony Juniper and Ian Skelly wrote *Harmony: A New Way of Looking at Our World* (2010). Attenborough's latest book *A Life on Our Planet* (2020) is presented as his witness statement and a vision for the future. His introduction to the book is titled "Our Greatest Mistake" in which he introduces the concept of how the biodiversity of the planet has been compromised by our actions. Much work is needed, with policy development, to prevent global warming and climate change is needed as a major factor in the potential deterioration of the life on earth. Everybody was excited by the Conference of the Parties (COP 24) Intergovernmental Panel on Climate Change Conference in Paris in 2016. Optimism created by scientists and politicians gave hope to the global community for a reduction climate change. This could be by changing industrial practices and lifestyle. However, the decision of the Trump Presidency to withdraw the USA from the agreement extinguished the hope of radical change. Fortunately, President Biden has a different view and optimism was reignited for the reorganised COP 26 meeting in Glasgow in December 2021. Bill Gates has just produced an important work *How to Avoid a Climate Disaster* (2021) in which he sets out a wide-ranging but accessible plan for how the world can get to zero greenhouse gas emissions in time to avoid a climate catastrophe. Emission reduction has been a key component of the COP meetings since they started in Rio de Janeiro in 1992, and trees are contributory factors in carbon capture leading to the REDD+ (Reduction of Emissions due to Deforestation and Forest Degradation) initiative. One-fifth of the world's population, 1.2 billion people, is dependent on forestry for their livelihoods. This is of particular significance in tropical countries and an activity which is being heavily compromised by illegal logging. In a paper to *Nature* in 2010, I argued that the only way to monitor deforestation is with satellite imagery and the application of stochastic models. International agencies, including the COP meetings, have been slow to come to consensus on international agreements for monitoring and reporting. Another unsatisfactory aspect is that the monitoring by earth observation which is done does not address the forest degradation that can result from environmental conditions such as wind or drought or from pests and diseases. Under such conditions, a forest can reach a tipping point from which trees do not recover and ultimately they die. This is possible to assess using non-linear mathematical modelling, but it is frustrating that there has been so little uptake of this approach to such an important global problem. Tipping point analysis of populations could also be relevant to the current pandemic in a very pessimistic scenario.

We humans are heavily dependent on food security generated by agriculture for their survival, and crops and animals can be subject to pandemics. Crops require suitable temperatures to grow and a fertile soil, which promotes the necessary nutrients and water, without being subject to toxins and growth retardants from pollution or adverse natural processes. This is compromised by climate change where some crops will not thrive at higher temperatures. For example, some of my early studies published in *Nature* investigated how fungi growing on straw in wet anaerobic soils could produce the growth hormone ethylene and retard root growth and crop productivity. Other studies showed how acetic acid could be produced by anaerobic bacteria under similar conditions and become toxic to seedlings. Another paper published in *Nature* showed how bacteria and fungi could cooperate to enhance fixation of nitrogen from the atmosphere and increase the supply of nitrogen as a nutrient to plants. Clearly, the value of microorganisms, particularly when they are close to roots (the rhizosphere), is a balance between beneficial and harmful effects. The community of microorganisms is now termed the microbiome. Microbiomes were first named for their interaction between plants and microorganisms, but subsequently, the term was applied to human and animal guts. Microbial ecology is the spine of this book, and the cover depicts a mixed population or microbiome of the human gut. Notable harmful organisms in the environment are the pathogens which can affect both roots and shoots of plants. However, it is often not recognised that some bacteria and fungi can effectively attack the pathogens and bring about the process of biological control. One route to achieve this is antibiosis. Indeed, Selman Waksman investigated antibiosis in a soil bacterium which led to the production of streptomycin, a discovery which resulted in a very important pharmaceutical and led to the award of the Nobel Prize. Preparation of biological control agents against pests and diseases for commercial delivery as a route to reduce the input of potentially harmful chemicals into the environment is an attractive option. In 1983 in a book *Soil Biotechnology*, I defined this new discipline as the study and manipulation of soil microorganisms and their processes to optimise crop productivity. This can be achieved by enhancing natural processes (augmentative) or by new introduction release to the ecosystem (inundative). In many ways, the uptake by industry has been disappointing, and this has in part been due to the agrochemical industry feeling threatened by the prospect of a reduced need for chemicals. There has also been concern because the public have sometimes thought of them as biological weapons which might spread disease in human populations. This is, even more, the case when the microorganisms or the plants with which they are associated have been genetically modified, attracting headlines in newspapers such as "Frankenstein Foods". In making the first UK release of a free-living genetically modified microorganism, created with my colleague Mark Bailey in Oxford, into soil, we were subjected to rigorous interrogation by government committees, and rightly so. Explaining such opportunities to the public became a huge challenge. It can be very useful to work with psychologists skilled at forming focus groups with the public to deliver messages and seek opinions with a view to developing trust. My colleague, Glynis Breakwell, has published a book in 2021 on *Mistrust* which is very relevant to pandemics.

When it was recognised by the early investigators that microorganisms could cause infection and spread of disease, and cause food to rot, there has often been a lack of recognition of the beneficial activities of microorganisms. A balanced view was presented by Bernard Dixon in his book *Power Unseen. How Microbes Rule the World* published in 1994. These benefits include degrading waste, providing nutrients and food products, and attacking pathogens, including bacteriophages in which viruses inactivate bacteria. A microbiologist is trained to show respect for microorganisms and work safely with aseptic procedures. There has also been the ongoing fear that microorganisms might be used offensively as weapons. Consequently, many countries have set up defence programmes to protect against this. At the time of the war in Iraq, it was believed that biological weapons posed a considerable threat and that, along with chemical weapons, was a justification for the invasion of Iraq. The media ran a story that such weapons were being produced at yogurt factory led by a woman they nicknamed Dr Death. I was immediately contacted because the woman had been one of our students and the security services wanted to know if I thought that possible. I thought it extremely unlikely. More importantly, the British weapons inspector Dr David Kelly who had made several official visits with the UN team to Iraq thought it very unlikely and he made that clear to the UK Government. That did not prevent the UK from supporting the invasion, and in mysterious circumstances, David Kelly took his own life as described in the books by Member of Parliament Norman Baker in 2007 *The Strange Death of David Kelly* following the enquiry by Lord Hutton and by Miles Goslett, *An Inconvenient Death* (2008), where he describes the conspiracy theories that resulted. Another conspiracy theory debate started with some of the early claims regarding the COVID-19 outbreak in Wuhan, China suggested that the virus could have escaped from the virology laboratory there, or that it had deliberately been released. The initial WHO team investigating these possibilities has indicated that both events are unlikely, but there will be ongoing investigation and debate. It is useful to consider the terms which define the spread of infection:

- **Endemic**: disease restricted to particular people in countries.
- **Outbreak**: greater than expected endemic in a single country or new area.
- **Epidemic**: outbreak that infects many people within a community or a region.
- **Pandemic**: an epidemic that has spread over multiple countries or countries.

Within months of the outbreak of COVID-19, the WHO declared a pandemic. Initial reactions by both politicians and scientists were that while recognising the seriousness of the situation control would be achieved as had happened with Ebola disease in Africa, which was an epidemic in recent times caused by another virus. Why has COVID-19 been so difficult to track and control? Many outbreaks of infection have been characterised by determining vectors of the disease. One of the earliest of these was Yellow Fever. The Cuban scientist Carlos J. Finlay showed that mosquitos spread the virus infection. The UNESCO Prize in Microbiology is named after him. With COVID-19, there has been no such suggestion of an insect vector, but the spread by animals, such as pangolins and bats, remains an open question. The threat of zoonotic diseases, which are relatively poorly understood, seems to be one of the big threats to mankind. Another complication in managing the disease is the frequency at which the virus can mutate, and the nature of the infection and potential to spread that the mutation can induce. Generally, these factors have been a far greater challenge than might have been anticipated, and certainly greater than is usually seen in bacterial diseases. Epidemiologists have produced widely different forecasts as the rate of infection but have produced some useful models to predict how bad the pandemic might become. It is disappointing, however, that there have been rather few assessments of how far the virus can move, and how atmospheric conditions indoors and outside might affect the spread. It is also not very clear how the virus can attach to different surfaces and how that influences infectivity. Although bacteria are generally easier to assess in these respects, largely stemming from the evolution of microbial ecology over the years, it should still have been possible to do more experimental studies with viruses to clarify their movement and attachment. When we released the genetically modified bacteria into the environment, it was necessary to monitor how far they spread and the impact on humans and biota generally. With COVID-19, it seems reasonable that the transmission could have been investigated in wind tunnels not just of droplets but of the virus itself in a controlled manner, providing better information on the risks of social mixing. Whereas in the past the ecology of viruses was challenging, modern techniques in molecular biology such as the polymerase chain reaction testing of infections have made ecological analysis far more straightforward.

It is also important to realise that pandemics can affect animals, the foot-and-mouth disease virus being a good example. From 1998 to 2001, the Pan Asia Strain affected Africa and Europe. Then, in 2001, another strain in the UK affected cloven-hoof animals, resulting in 6 million sheep and cattle being killed to try to halt the spread at a cost of £86 million to the UK. The cause was almost certainly infected waste meat getting into the supply chain and extensive distribution across the country. It was both an animal and human tragedy at huge cost to farming families both emotionally and financially. The impact of the disease to the management of farming and the environment prompted an examination of both farming practices and the psychosocial effects of such a disaster, justifying the need for a holistic approach.

As the COVID-19 pandemic spread, it became clear that the only effective route to deal with the problem was immunisation. The first Briton to win the Carlos J. Finlay Prize was Cesar Milstein for his immunological work developing monoclonal antibodies, which also gained him the 1984 Nobel Prize in Physiology or Medicine. Monoclonal antibodies are today potentially valuable to work against certain cancers. However, that is potential cure rather than prevention. Globally, teams have been working on a variety of approaches using inactivated virus, protein subunits, messenger RNA, and adenovirus (common cold virus) vectors, made possible by the rapid advancement of molecular biology, and there has been an amazing degree of success. Much of that has been due to the excellence of the science but also to the pragmatic approach to registration which in normal circumstances would have taken far longer.

Politically and bioethically, a decision had to be taken on the priority for vaccination. In the UK, it was decided that age was a key factor in determining risk of serious illness or death, as well as front-line medical and care workers, and priorities for vaccination were set on that basis. Even though young people and their teachers are at lower risk, there could have been an argument that they were more deserving of protection. It is also critical that vaccination is rolled out in the developing world to prevent health inequality globally. Decisions were taken using the scientific and medical evidence, and there is little obvious indication that ethics were considered. Ben Bramble considered these issues in his book *Pandemic Ethics* (2020) which he generously made available by open-access on-line. Many of the issues discussed in the present book have bioethical implications. For example, the use of genetic engineering whether for human or environmental benefit has already been mentioned, and this has usually been considered by the Nuffield Council on Bioethics and other regulatory bodies. Bioethics is an important part of moral theology. Theological issues have already been mentioned in getting the ideas of Galileo Galilei and Pierre Teilhard de Chardin accepted by the Church. Charles Darwin also struggled in getting his ideas on evolution accepted by the Church. Richard Dawkins in his recent book *Outgrowing God* (2019) has described the beauty of classical and molecular evolution and indicated that God was not necessary for such creation. However, neither does he present an alternative for the primary trigger for cosmological or biological routes to our origin. The alternative view especially how it relates to the pandemic is put eloquently by John Lennox in his book *Where Is God in a Coronavirus World* (2020). Even though Stephen Hawking was not a practising Christian, he did admit the possibility of a God to create life. He pointed out that God is bound by the Uncertainty Principle in physics and cannot know both the speed and the position of a particle. He continues to say that all the evidence points to God being an inveterate gambler, who throws the dice on every possible occasion!

We cannot ignore the role of organised religion in conserving the environment and communities. Communities without organised religious beliefs, such as those in Amazonia and the aboriginal people in Australia, should be brought into such debates.

I have found such communities very helpful to engage with. On a visit to Eastern Australia on behalf of the Organisation for Economic Co-operation and Development (OECD), I met with aboriginal leaders who value land highly and were concerned about sugar cane farmers applying so much nitrogen fertiliser that it was leaching into groundwaters and flowing out to sea to damage the Great Barrier Reef. They were right!

It was a great privilege for 17 years to be coordinator of the OECD Co-operative Research Programme on Biological Resource Management for Sustainable Agricultural Systems for which I was awarded the OBE, and to receive the Carlos J. Finlay Prize for work on the soil microbiome during my tenure as Chair of the Biology Commission of the International Society of Soil Science. The main reflection I am left with during the pandemic revolves around the topic of sustainability. My colleague Tim Jackson wrote a book *Prosperity without Growth* (2009) in which he showed that the finite resources of our planet can be effectively managed economically, in line with OECD goals which I support. The United Nations Environment Programme produced an excellent set of 17 Sustainable Development Goals with 169 targets and 244 indicators. Some progress is being made in achieving them by various routes. For example, some of these can be tracked from space using satellite imagery. However, in many arenas such as carbon emissions, progress is slow. Yet pandemic with its lockdowns has resulted in some improvements, such as a reduction in transport emissions. It has also made us consider if it is sensible to allow some Asian animal markets to operate as they do. Not only do they compromise the maintenance of biodiversity, but they are also a potential vector for the spread of disease. Sustainability would increase with a greater emphasis on vegan diets, both from more efficient food production systems but also by reducing greenhouse gas emissions from animals. There is also the opportunity to use more biofuel as a renewable source of energy, provided that it has a satisfactory life cycle assessment and does not compromise environmental resources. There has been great consistency of thought in preserving the planet by people such as Pope Francis and Jim Lovelock who come from such different perspectives, and all religions as well as atheists like Richard Dawkins have much to contribute to the debates. As we have seen scientific method and analysis has always had debate at its heart since the challenge by the Catholic Church to the views of Galileo Galilei on the nature of the planets. The Bishop of Kingston, Richard Cheetham, has spearheaded the Anglican position on the relationship of science and theology. We must be inclusive to all views for debate, be up to the challenge of today's problems, and develop a path to a sustainable world of global landscapes in which we can all flourish and be healthy.

As I neared the completion of the manuscript for this book in the summer of 2021, I was given a book by the Nobel Prize winner Paul Nurse *What Is Life?* He describes three principles of life:

1. The ability to evolve through natural selection.
2. Life forms are bounded by physical entities. They are separated from, but in communication with, their environments.
3. Living entities are chemical, physical, and informational machines. They construct their own metabolism and use it to maintain themselves, grow and reproduce.

He writes as a geneticist and cell biologist who has worked on how the reproduction of cells is controlled. He points out that for every one of the 30 trillion or more human cells in our bodies, there is at least one microbial cell. He also reminds us that viruses are not cells as such but chemical entities with a genome based on DNA or RNA with the capacity to make the coat protein which encapsulates them. Nothing in his book is inconsistent with the views in this book which I have written as a microbiologist with a primary interest in the environment. I will, however, try to extend the discussion to the sustainability of life from scientific, social, and moral perspectives and suggest that we should be optimistic to secure our future by deploying science effectively in policy and governance. In writing, I have used information in the books cited in the bibliography and in the scientific and popular press. However, the views expressed are mine, whether they are consistent or not with those that I have read.

Please note that the black and white images in this book are all available to download for free, in full colour, via the Support Materials tab on the book's webpage at https://www.routledge.com/9781032303888

2 Cosmology and Quantum Biology

We live on a hunk of rock and metal that is one of 400 billion other stars that make up the Milky Way Galaxy which is one of billions of other galaxies which make up a universe which may be one of a very large number, perhaps infinite number, of other universes. That is a perspective on human life and our culture that is well worth pondering.

Carl Sagan 1934–1996.

The more I study nature, the more I stand amazed at the work of the Creator. Science brings men nearer to God.

Louis Pasteur 1822–1895

Cosmology is the science of the origin and development of the universe. Modern cosmology is dominated by the Big Bang Theory, which brings together observational astronomy and particle physics. One of the most readable accounts of the story of cosmic evolution, science, and civilisation is by Carl Sagan (1981) *Cosmos*. He describes 15 billion years of cosmic evolution which has transformed matter and life into consciousness and made an acclaimed television series based on the book where he makes his ideas comprehensible and exciting. One feature of the book is the stimulating and thought-provoking multiple quotations at the start of each chapter. His primary approach is from that of an astronomer. One of the most important early astronomers was the Italian scientist Galileo Galilei (1564–1642) who was Professor of Mathematics at the University of Pisa. Galilei was forced by the Catholic Church under threat of torture to recant his heretical view that the earth moved about the Sun (heliocentric) and not *vice versa* (geocentric), being forced to remain under house arrest. However, it is not always recognised that Galileo overplayed his hand in that his two proofs of the earth's motion (based on tides and on sunspots) were, in fact, not valid. So even though Galileo's discoveries in astronomy were truly epoch-making, it highlights the nature of conjecture in science which is commonly how evidence evolves. From Pisa he accepted a professorship at the University of Leiden and, in 1638, wrote a book *Discorsi* in 1638 which describes materials science and kinematics and regarded as the foundation of modern physics. It was published by the company Elsevier in Leiden, a company that is still at the forefront of scientific publishing. It took until 1979 for Pope John Paul II to cautiously reverse the condemnation of Galileo by the Holy Inquisition 346 years earlier.

The Enlightenment which ran from 1715 to 1789 was an intellectual and philosophical movement. It was during this time that the telescope was developed, particularly in Holland. Light was key to the time, and it was then that the microscope was also developed, linking the very large to the very small. At the centre of the activity

DOI: 10.1201/9781003304845-2

was Antonie van Leeuwenhoek. With his crude microscope which had been developed to examine the quality of cloth, he discovered in a drop of water 'animalcules' which we now understand to be microbes. With his colleague Christiaan Huygens, he also saw human sperm cells, key in the understanding of human reproduction. The microbes were detected in boiled water and Huygens proposed that they must have colonised the water from the air, overturning the concept of spontaneous generation which could have arisen. It took a further two centuries for Louis Pasteur to prove the speculation correct. Leeuwenhoek and Huygens can, therefore, be regarded as the fathers of the germ theory of disease, so important to modern medicine, even though they originally had no practical motives in mind. Sagan emphasises the importance of optics in studying the cosmos and in his chapter on the lives of stars he quotes from Isaac Newton (1642–1727) in his book *Optics* 'God is able to create particles of matter of several sizes and figures ... and perhaps of different densities and forces, and thereby to vary the laws of nature, and make worlds of several sorts in several parts of the universe. At least I find nothing of contradiction in all this'.

Stephen Hawking was a leading theoretical physicist and cosmologist, serving as the Lucasian Professor of Mathematics, as had Newton, in the University of Cambridge from 1979 to 2009. It is interesting how often the subjects of Cosmology, Physics, and Mathematics converge in job functions. At the centre of much of his work has been the black hole, a region of spacetime where gravity is so strong that nothing, including particles and electromagnetic radiation such as light, can escape from. Albert Einstein had predicted their existence when he published his theory of relativity in 1916. It was first spotted in 1964 in the Cygnus constellation 6070 light years away and Hawking showed that they emit radiation which can be detected. However, in his book *A Brief History of Time: From the Big Bang to Black Holes* (1988), his suggestion that radiation of spontaneously created particle-antiparticle pairs is incorrect. The Nobel Prize for Physics was shared in 2020 by Roger Penrose from Oxford University for his work proving that black holes could and should form in the universe. The topological picture used in the proof is the foundation of general relativity. The impact of Hawking's work is best seen in his last book *Brief Answers to the Big Questions* (2018), completed by his daughter Lucy shortly after his death. Few people would question the ten big questions he selected for an answer, but they would not necessarily agree with the answers provided.

1. Is there a God?

    The universe was spontaneously created out of nothing, according to the laws of science. However, he would accept the laws of science as God, but it would not be a personal God that you would meet and put questions to. If, however, there were a personal God, he would ask if he had thought of M-theory in 11 dimensions. He does not believe in an afterlife, but that we live on by passing our genes to our children.

2. How did it all begin?

    M-theory predicts that a great many universes were created out of nothing. The beginning of the universe itself in the Hot Big Bang is the ultimate high-energy laboratory for testing M-theory. This could all end in a Big

Crunch when too much matter in the universe starts falling towards each other. This could be 20 billion years in the future!

3. Is there other intelligent life in the universe?

If there is intelligent life elsewhere in the universe, it must have been a very long way away; otherwise, it would probably have visited us by now. However, it might have been overlooked. No obvious possibilities provide a satisfactory answer to the question.

4. Can we predict the future?

Astronomy was the first science to be developed but the analysis of quantum behaviour is important for determinism. Laplace put forward the view that the motion of particles was completely determined provided that the positions and speeds are known at one time. However, Werner Heisenberg in his Uncertainty Principle said that these could not be known accurately. Even limited predictability might be removed in the light of black holes.

5. What is inside a black hole?

Black holes are characterised by their overall mass, electric charge, and spin outside the event horizon, but the event horizon itself contains information needed to tell us what has fallen into the black hole in a way that goes beyond these three characteristics the black hole has. As particles escape from the black hole, the hole will lose mass and shrink, increasing the rate of emission of particles.

6. Is time travel possible?

Rapid space travel and travel back in time cannot be ruled out according to our current thinking. It would create great logical problems, but there is great hope in the unifying form of string theory, M-theory.

7. Will we survive on earth?

An asteroid collision would be a threat against which we have no defence. However, the last was about 66 million years ago and killed the dinosaurs. The most immediate threat is runaway climate change, releasing carbon dioxide and melting ice caps. Our climate could become like that of Venus with a temperature of 250°C.

8. Should we colonise space?

Within the next hundred years, we will be able to travel to anywhere in the solar system, except maybe the outer planets which might take 500 years. This is to be welcomed.

9. Will artificial intelligence outsmart us?

Our future is a race between the growing power of our technology and the wisdom with which we use it. Wisdom needs to prevail and not fall into the trap when the computer was asked if there is a God and the computer responded by saying there is now and promptly fused the plug!

10. How do we shape the future?

Nuclear fusion would become a practical power source and would provide us with an inexhaustible supply of clean energy, without pollution or global warming, facilitating a switch to electric cars.

The previous book by Stephen Hawking, written with Leonard Mlodinow in 2010, *The Grand Design: New Answers to the Ultimate Questions of Life*, explained the thoughts about model-dependent realism and about the multiverse concept of reality in which there are many universes. This was once the province of philosophers but is now where scientists, philosophers, and theologians meet. The Stoics, a third-century school of Greek philosophy, distinguished between human statutes and natural laws, the latter including obedience to parents and veneration to God. The Christian philosopher St. Thomas Aquinas (1225–1275) argued for the existence of God in this way, saying 'it is clear that inanimate bodies reach their end, not by chance but by intention ... There is therefore an intelligent personal being by whom everything in nature is ordered to its end'. The philosopher who was an architect of the rule of law of nature was Rene Descartes (1596–1650). He believed that all physical phenomena must be explained in terms of collisions of moving masses and the laws were the precursors of Newton's laws of motion. They did not imply that the bodies had minds. The laws depended on a set of initial conditions. With the existence of such laws, there were attempts to reconcile them with the concept of God. He said that God could at will alter the truth or falsity of ethical propositions or mathematical theorems but not nature. He believed that God ordained the laws of nature but had no choice in them as they were the only possible laws. He argued that this did not impinge on God's authority, but they were governed by God's own intrinsic nature. Essentially when God set the world in motion, he left it entirely alone, according to Descartes. A similar position was adopted by Isaac Newton (1643–1727). Newton believed that the solar system did not arise out of chaos by the laws of nature. Instead, he believed that God created it and conserved it in the same state and condition and was conserved by him. Three questions arise on the laws: (1) What is the origin? (2) Are there exceptions such as miracles? and (3) Is there only one possible set? Kepler (1571–1630), Galileo (1564–1642), Descartes, and Newton were all affirmative on the first question. Opinions on the second question have been divided. Plato (428–348 BC) and Aristotle (384–322 BC) held that there can be no exceptions. Most Christian thinkers argued that God must be able to suspend the laws to accomplish miracles and Newton was in that camp. On the third question Aristotle and Plato believed, like Descartes and later Einstein (1879–1955), that the principles of nature exist out of necessity as they are the only ones that make logical sense. Aristotle felt that laws could be derived but Galileo modified this by applying them only to what nature did rather than what it ought to do. If we accept that God created the universe, the question remains who created God. In that view, the entity of first cause argument is the creator is God, although there are those who argue that science can explain all without the involvement of a divine being. The argument is that spontaneous creation is the reason there is something rather than nothing, why the universe exists, and why we exist.

A very elegant analysis and dismissal of Hawking and Mlodinow's views on God are provided by David Bentley Hart, an Eastern Orthodox scholar of religion and philosopher in his book *The Experience of God. Being, Consciousness and Bliss*, published in 2013. He argues that the Hawking's multiverses generated by quantum fluctuations do not have a role for God has not much to do with God anyway and is a false conclusion drawn from a confused question. Hawking views God only as a demiurge, coming after the law of gravity but before the present universe, and allowing spontaneous generation and creation. Hawking does not allow that the concept of God might concern a reality not temporarily prior to this or that world, but logically necessarily prior to all worlds, all physical laws, all quantum events, and even all possibilities of laws and events. Under classical metaphysics, Hawking and Mlodinow miss the point of creation because it would be just as necessary if only physical laws and states existed without an ordered universe. When properly conceived, God is not a force or cause within nature, nor a kind of supreme natural explanation. The multiverse concept as an alternative to God as described by Hawking and Mlodinow is clearly wrong as if there is a multiverse, there is a vacuum from which universes pop in and out of existence, but a vacuum is not nothing in physics, it is something. For example, it carries energy so someone must have created it as the first cause. Maybe the universe is cyclic (an argument often used to avoid the idea of creation), and if it has always existed, there is something rather than nothing, and if there is something, there is a source for it.

It remains a question as to when the Big Bang took place but modelling of such events is a possibility. To produce a good model, Stephen Hawking believes that it should satisfy four criteria: (1) elegance, (2) few arbitrary or adjustable elements, (3) agree with and explain all existing observation, and (4) make detailed predictions about future observations. The Christian philosopher St. Augustine (354–430) said that time was a property of the world that was created by God and that time did not exist before that creation as his model. Aristotle believed the world was made of the elements earth, air, fire, and water, with no adjustable elements. His theories often did not make definite predictions, but when they were made, they were not always in agreement with observations. This should not really surprise us because similar inconsistencies can occur in modern science as models are tested by improved collection of information. This is the excitement of science as it evolves towards a complete understanding of the universe. For example, dark matter is thought to account for about 85% of the matter in the universe, and in a report in *Nature* in May 2021, cosmologists used a sophisticated megapixel camera between 2013 and 2019 in the southern sky to map its presence in the universe and produce the most-detailed 3D cosmic map of the universe's history.

Hawking pointed out that there is great hope in string theory. The book *Superstrings. A Theory of Everything* by Paul Davies and Julian Brown published in 1988 spelt out the opportunity to unify physics and develop a unified theory of all forces of nature. The theory is that the physical world is made up of nothing but little strings. It is based on physics, but nothing is beyond its scope in discipline coverage. The argument is that everything, including all biological and chemical systems, is dictated by the laws of physics and nothing else. It is based on the philosophy of reductionism. In this view, psychology is reduced to biology, biology is reduced to chemistry, and chemistry to physics. However, it is unreasonable to expect it to understand many complex features. For example, the work of Galileo and Newton leading to atomic theory was supported by the elucidation of the laws of motion for material bodies, showing that the movement of atoms obeys physical laws that led to Laplace producing his demon calculator as one of the first attempts to produce a Theory of Everything. However, no attempt was made in this to explain why the universe contains the atoms it does. The nature of forces between atoms was also vague, as was time and space between the forces. It was regarded that space and time were there but not part of physics. It has taken very much longer for physicists to identify the level of structure that underlies this physical richness. The quantum theory of Max Planck began with the suggestion that electromagnetic radiation comes only in distinct packets, or quanta, which we term photons. Quantum mechanics can be observed quite simply in the 'double slit experiment'. If light is shone through a pair of slits, then the emerging light will illuminate a series of light and dark bands on the screen. The bands are known as interference patterns. They show the wave nature of light when light passes through both slits to emerge as two beams that recombine to reinforce each other or cancel each other out. Relativity theory relinquishes notions about space, time, and motion and replaces the intuitive physics of Newton. Quantum theory is an equally radical reappraisal of ideas about the nature of matter. We shall see later that this is very important in biology. The book edited by Davies and Brown invites many distinguished physicists to outline the scope of superstrings. Some of the optimism expressed by Hawking and Davies and Brown are tempered in the book by John Barrow *Theories of Everything. The Quest for Ultimate Explanation* (1990). He claims to put a more reasonable perspective on how long it might take to come up with such a theory, if ever. He also spells out the input of Roger Boscovich (1711–1787) to the first visionary of the Theory of Everything in his book in 1758 *Theoria Philosophiae Naturalis*. Boscovich was a Dalmatian Jesuit, poet and architectural advisor to Popes, cosmopolitan diplomat and man of affairs, socialite and theologian, confidant of governments, and Fellow of the Royal Society, but most of all a mathematician and scientist. He extended the overall picture of Newton in several ways and sought to derive all observed physical phenomena from a single law. He showed that nature was composed of identical elementary particles and showed larger objects in nature with finite sizes was a consequence of the way their elementary constituents interact one with another.

In June 2021, the London Institute of Mathematical Sciences compiled a list of the 23 most important mathematical questions of our time. At the top of the list was **Theory of Everything**. Will this be resolved by string theory, loop quantum gravity, or something new? Also included in the list was **Thermodynamics of Life**. According to Darwin's theory, evolution is the result of mutation, selection, and inheritance, but from a physical perspective, we do not understand how life got started in the first place. What is the thermodynamic basis for emergent self-selection and adaptation of which biology is just one instance? Can it be used to create digital artificial life? **Theory of Immortality**. Ageing is ascribed to the accumulation of errors – an inevitable consequence of the increase of disorder. But mounting experimental evidence suggests that ageing is not a fact of life. Is it a thermodynamics necessity, or is it instead favoured by natural selection? Can we mathematically describe the pros and cons of ageing? Is it possible to slow or even stop it?

The recent text by Michio Kaku, *The God Equation. The Quest for a Theory of Everything* (2021), is a very readable update on the way the Theory of Everything has developed. He points out that the final form of string theory has yet to be revealed and therefore it is premature to compare it to the present universe. In some respects, the theory is going backwards, revealing new mathematics and concepts along the way. As we do not yet know the final fundamental principles, we cannot compare it with experiment. My view is that we should not be despondent because this is following the path of normal scientific investigation. He nevertheless goes into arguments on God like Hawking and Einstein. Albert Einstein wrote a thought-provoking work translated into English in 1935 *The World as I See It*. Kaku quotes Einstein 'God does not play dice with the world', meaning that not everything can be reduced to chance and uncertainty. He adds that Hawking said that 'Sometimes God throws the dice where you cannot find them', meaning that dice may land in black holes where laws of the quantum may not hold. He also said that the Big Bang took place in an instant of time such that there was not enough time for God to create the universe as we know it. Kaku's teacher at school said that God also loved the earth that he put it just to the right of the Sun. This was not too close, or the oceans would boil and not too far or the oceans would freeze! With about 4000 planets orbiting other stars which are not close enough to support life. We are on a planet which sustains intelligent life and so perhaps there is a loving God after all. In the multiverse theory put forward by Kaku, our universe is just a bubble amongst coexisting bubble universes which are being created all the time. On this basis, time might not have started with the Big Bang, but at a time before the beginning of our universe. The totality of universes could be eternal but that still opens the question of the existence of God. Theologians have tried to use logic to prove the existence of God. St Thomas Aquinas and set out three potential proofs of relevance to our thinking:

1. **Cosmological proof**: God is the First Mover to set the universe in motion.
2. **Teleological proof**: God was the First Designer of objects of great complexity and sophistication.
3. **Ontological proof**: The most perfect being imaginable is God. If God did not exist, he would not be perfect and therefore he must exist.

Kant challenged ontological proof because perfection and existence are separate and to be perfect does not imply that something must exist. Teleological proof could be driven by evolution and a First Designer is not necessary. Cosmological proof is less clear and a possible logical consequence of a Theory of Everything, but where did that come from. At that point, physics becomes metaphysics. Therefore, the questions of St. Thomas Aquinas remain today. However, we should not just think of Christianity where God created the world in an instant of time. For example, in Buddhism there is no God. The universe had no beginning or end, only timeless Nirvana. A multiverse theory could approach this contradiction. In these religions, as well as others, we also should consider the influence of the important human aspect of faith.

It is quantum mechanics, initiated by Max Planck in 1900, that would challenge everything we knew about the universe. Roger Penrose extended his work on the application of quantum mechanics and black holes to the analysis mind. The mind has occupied philosophers for centuries and perhaps one of the most famous philosophical statements is *Cogito ergo sum* (I think therefore I am) by the seventeenth-century philosopher Rene Descartes. He believed that science would establish objective truth as being self-evident and that there was a certainty in scientific knowledge not being found in other branches of reality. He argued that scientists can deduce the phenomena of nature through the various branches of mathematics. Penrose's book published in 1989 *The Emperor's New Mind: Concerning Computers, Minds, and the Laws of Physics* encapsulates this thinking and was followed by a sequel in 1994 *Shadows of the Mind: A Search for the Missing Science of Consciousness*. He argued that human consciousness is non-algorithmic and therefore cannot be modelled on a conventional Turing machine, including a digital computer. In this respect, human thinking can never be replaced by a machine. Although quantum physics plays an important role in consciousness, the collapse of quantum wavefunction is important in brain function. Some critics have said this is speculative and Penrose agrees! It would also cast some doubt on the use of artificial intelligence and machine learning, two arenas that are advancing rapidly at present. Nevertheless, it need not be inconsistent as Penrose is addressing the mind as such which is far more complex that the machines used in machine learning and artificial intelligence. He also concedes that the new science may eventually explain the physical basis of the mind. In *Shadows of the Mind*, he uses the Incompleteness Theorem of Kurt Godel (1906–1978), which is stated as:

> For any computable axiomatic (postulate or assumption taken as true for further reasoning and argument) that is powerful enough to describe the arithmetic of natural numbers (used for counting and ordering) that
>
> 1. If a logical or axiomatic system is omega-consistent (avoiding combinations which are intuitively contradictory), it cannot be syntactically (with respect to every formula) complete.
> 2. The consistency of axioms cannot be proved within their own systems.

Godel was a theist in the Christian tradition and believed that God is personal, and philosophy is rationalistic, idealistic, optimist, and theological. Penrose, in line with so many scientists, declares he has an agnostic persuasion but has always in an open-minded manner been keen to develop metaphysical arguments. He entered an online debate with the Christian philosopher William Lane Craig, an advocate that theism is a unifying force of reality, in The Big Conversation on Christian Radio on 4 October 2019. Penrose reiterated that maths is discovered and not invented, and that a metaphysical vision of philosophy is reality and is not dead. He declared three worlds: (1) physical, (2) mental, and (3) abstract. The physical is necessary according to Penrose, and the mental, including morality and aesthetics, is necessary according to Craig. Most mystery is in the abstract. Penrose declared that much of divinity is too vague for him to understand but would be open to any evidence which would allow him an afterlife. Most metaphysical hypothesis cannot be investigated but only postulated. Craig indicated that such postulation is in line with the thinking of the Athenian philosopher Plato who was the father of idealism which was elitist but a theory of reality. He thought that in ethics and moral philosophy a good life requires a certain kind of knowledge. A meeting attended by Penrose in the Vatican aired a view that an infinite collection of aeons (long spans of geological time) is created by God, and that fine-tuning facilitated life in the universe or multiverses. Penrose admits not being able to understand this. In Penrose's thinking, it seems to me that his analysis of the mind in quantum terms supports his agnostic view on the physical aspects, but in the mental and abstract views, the existence of God could be justified by faith, which is the choice of the individual, especially in the light that proof is extremely unlikely. In *Shadows of the Mind*, Penrose examines cytoskeletons and microtubules, minute substructures that lie deep within the brain's neurons. He considers that microtubules, rather than the neurons, might be the basic units of the brain. Within in them the collective quantum effects necessary for consciousness reside. This would affect the philosophical viewpoint on reality.

The views of Penrose on the involvement of quantum theory on the biological function of the mind can potentially be applied to all living organisms. An approach to this was put powerfully by Johnjoe McFadden in his book *Quantum Evolution* published in 2000. As a molecular microbiologist, he reminds us that living cells are controlled by DNA. Physics tell us that single molecules are controlled by quantum mechanics rather than classical laws. Particles behave the same as light in quantum mechanics. Single atoms fired through slits generate the same type of interference patterns as light, which is well understood within standard quantum mechanics. Fundamental particles can be in more than one universe at the same time as parallel universes. However, this coexistence is itself wavy and for bulky objects which may have billions of particles the peaks and troughs tend to average to zero and cancel each other out. However, if there are, for example, electrons in some parallel universe, they will not be able to interact with those in our universe and we will never know of their existence. Every living organism is controlled by DNA which is not barred from quantum behaviour, just as are the fullerenes or 'buckyballs' of 60 carbon atoms in a cage structure for which the Nobel Prize in Chemistry was awarded to Robert Curl, Harold Kroto, and Richard Smalley in 1996. In the past, it is odd that this has not been explored fully. Quantum mechanics gives cells the ability to initiate specific actions, including mutations, very important in the current context of the COVID-19 virus mutations. This is probably a fundamental aspect of life and is the central feature of evolution, providing variation which is honed by natural selection into evolutionary paths. It may also help in understanding how life began and any small primordial path could generate life by access to the quantum multiverse. It challenges some of the evolutionary theories such as Darwinism where evolution is random but instead is directed over the past 4 billion years. Cells may be able to mutate specific genes and provide an advantage in the environment in which they exist. Quantum evolution must be at the centre of consciousness and free will, as implied by Penrose. It also gives a better view of how to understand life and death. It was exciting for me to be able to talk with my colleague Johnjoe McFadden as these concepts emerged but also at an early stage, he engaged our quantum physicist colleague at the University of Surrey, Jim Al-Khalili. Together they wrote a sequel book *Life on the Edge. The Coming Age of Quantum Biology* in 2014. They examine some of life's puzzles such as how do migrating birds know where to go? How do we smell the scent of a rose? How do our genes copy themselves with such precision? All seem to be rooted in the quantum world. McFadden's research in the past has been to examine the genes of bacteria that cause tuberculosis and meningitis. These diseases must surely be under the same principles of genetic evolution, but surely so must be the genetic variants of the COVID-19 virus in the current pandemic.

3 Origins of Life

How you'd exalt if I could put you back
  Six hundred years, blot out cosmogeny, geology and ethnology, what not....
  And yet set you square with Genesis again.

Robert Browning 1812–1889

There is a grandeur in this view of life, with its several powers, having been originally breathed into a few forms or into one; and that while this planet has gone cycling on according to the fixed law of gravity, from so simple a beginning endless life forms most beautiful and most wonderful have been, and are being, evolved.

Charles Darwin 1809–1882

The preceding chapter set out the physical framework for the development of life on the planet. In this chapter, I will start by providing aspects of the palaeontological evidence of life from the fossil record. Palaeontology not only involves primarily geology and biology but also exploits mathematics and engineering. I will then move to analysing the chemical markers and the events which may have led to their genesis. The markers are largely contained in the geological shales and cherts of the Cambrian and Pre-Cambrian Period (Figure 3.1).

Human palaeontology is the most recent of the eras studied but does not normally include modern man (*Homo sapiens*) who evolved about 0.2 million years ago from ancient man (*Homo erectus*) who evolved about 2 million years ago, and apes prior to that about 6 million years ago. The Pleistocene period from 2.5 million to 0.1 million years ago covers this period of evolution. Pierre Teilhard de Chardin (1881–1955), a Jesuit priest, was an important human palaeontologist who discovered remains of early man at Chou Kou Tien in 1927. He wrote a book *The Phenomenon of Man* in 1955, giving rise to conflicts with the Catholic Church mentioned in Chapter 1. The book is essentially a scientific and philosophical exploration of the evolutionary process in nature. Man is the product of this evolution, but he differs from other products in that he is conscious of it and an active agent in it. In that respect, it could be linked to Penrose's views on the mind. The three stages of evolution he recognises are the chemical, the organic, and the psychosocial. The three main stages are separation and consolidation of the earth itself, appearance of life on earth, and the appearance of thought or the ability to reflect. The rise in consciousness is an increase in knowledge or in life. This could not appear suddenly and there must have been some preparation, including inorganic particles containing pre-life components. He also considered that there are two types of energy. Tangential energy is that which corresponds with physical energy such as electrical energy. The other he called radial energy which is important to the third stage of evolution and corresponds with spiritual energy. He describes life being multiplied by reproduction so that it could spread.

DOI: 10.1201/9781003304845-3

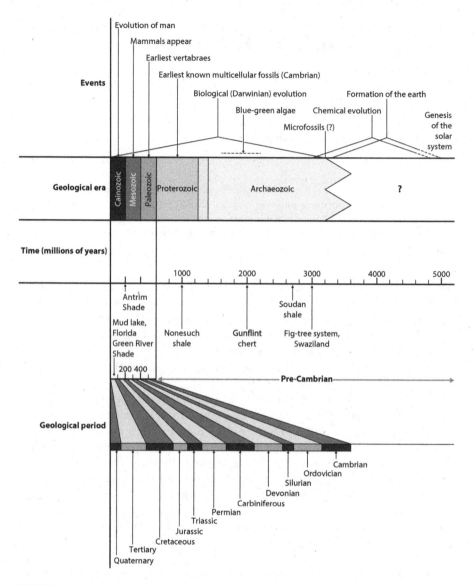

FIGURE 3.1   Geological timescale.

Conjugation or the union of cells led to the formation of more complex beings and evolution to move upwards. The fossil record shows many illustrations of the appearance of new phyla in this way. The primates that are linked to man gained ever more complex nervous systems, including a brain to increase consciousness. The next step for man is thought and reflection which Teilhard termed hominisation. He also used the term noosphere to describe the layer of thought to spread around the world. Survival is not by isolation but by collectivism, allowing each person to develop. At the centre of this is the Omega point. To develop truth must be sought in a unified and organised way. Psychology supports the spiritual side of man, and this is where science and religion can connect. In Teilhard's case, this is through Christianity.

So, with man at the summit of the evolutionary tree, when and where did the first living systems originate? The Phanerozoic timescale which was the first 600 million years has been well-documented and is divided into eras, periods, and epochs from stratigraphical dating and from the fossils themselves. Evidence for the Pre-Cambrian (the oldest) period came later. Most of the dating is done using isotopic measurements. The fossils are the results of living organisms, and much attention has been on the prokaryotic blue-green algae (cyanobacteria) leaving calcareous residues of their mats as they settled. Other bacteria also existed, and these can be seen in cherts (sedimentary rocks composed almost entirely of silica with the general properties of quartz). The structures seen in the rocks often resemble those of organisms in soils today. For example, at Harlech Castle in Wales, an organism that requires ammonia has been found bearing a resemblance to those in older rocks, thought to be enriched from a continuous input of urea from human action! The oldest such rock is the Fig Tree Chert from South Africa at 3100 million years (Figure 3.1). Much younger are the shales (about 60 million years old) which are sedimentary rocks formed from mud with clay and silt. The challenge has been to evaluate if there are chemical markers in the ancient rocks which have analogues in modern organisms. As I investigated such processes during my postgraduate studies referred to in Chapter 1, I was stimulated by the treatise produced at that time by Nobel Laureate Melvin Calvin on *Chemical Evolution* in 1969. To assemble a cell, critical building molecules are amino acids, polypeptides, purines, pyrimidines, and nucleotides, which would have to come from the primordial atmosphere of methane, ammonia, and water. Of greatest interest in determining markers has been the lipid fraction and especially those with distinctive branched carbon chain structures contained in the lipid (fat) fraction, notably phytane (17 carbon atoms) and pristane (18 carbon atoms). Both are thought to be derived from chlorophyll, the green photosynthetic pigment. Importantly pristane is formed in sediments on oxidising conditions and phytane is formed under reducing conditions. The ratio is therefore an indicator of the oxidative status of sediments. The cellular equivalent of these markers is isoprenoid, which can then be polymerised to squalene (30 carbon atoms), and then can potentially be cyclised into steroids and triterpenoids. We saw in the Introduction that these have been found in a methane-utilising bacterium and the fully saturated steranes and triterpanes found in ancient sediments. Much attention in the field of study has been the photosynthetic bacteria or blue-green algae, and green algae, but the important factor seems be whether the cells have internal membrane networks which are important sources of lipids.

The principal investigation on the chemical origin on Earth was carried out by Stanley Miller, supervised by Harold Urey, in 1952 at the University of Chicago. The experiments used methane, ammonia, and hydrogen, thought to be the primeval atmosphere on Earth, sealed in a 5 L glass container, and connected to a smaller flask which was half-full of water, which was heated, and the water vapour allowed to enter the larger flask. Lightening was simulated from electrical sparks generated by electrodes. The atmosphere was then cooled, and the condensate allowed to run into a U-shaped trap. One day later, the solution in the trap was pink and after a week, it was deep red and turbid. After removing the flask and adding mercuric chloride to prevent contamination, barium peroxide and sulphuric acid were used to stop the reaction. Following evaporation, paper chromatography was used to identify the amino acids glycine, alpha-alanine, and bet-alanine, with less certainty on aspartic acid and alpha-amino-butyric acid. The chemistry involved the formation of hydrogen cyanide and formaldehyde as intermediates. This overall reaction showed that the simple amino acids, which are the building blocks of proteins, can be formed from the primeval gas atmosphere induced by the electric spark energy. The question is whether the amino acids generated could have been nucleobases for the creation of RNA as the basic building block of life. Although subsequent investigations on the 1952 samples and other new experiments in 2008 and 2010 have shown that additional amino acids formed, there has been very limited success on even identification of the intermediate peptides which would have been necessary. Although the experiments are very interesting, no proof has been obtained on this abiogenic route to life.

Most texts on the origin of life have discussed the Miller-Urey experiments with the same conclusions. One such text published in 2005 by Robert Hazen *Genesis. The Scientific Quest for Life's Origin* approaches gives his perspective as a geophysicist and astrobiologist at the Carnegie Institute in Washington, DC. He rejects the 'primordial soup' concept in the Miller-Urey experiments as irrelevant because the soup was too dilute and had too many molecular species which could not contribute to life. He points out that a mixture of elements is found near deep-ocean vents at crushing pressures and high temperatures. Life might have started in such a place, nourished by the mineralised organics, and energised by the geochemical forces on the surface of the earth, ocean waves, and lapping rocky shores. He discusses the relevance of laboratory and field observations but indicates that natural processes exist beyond what we now know or what we can comprehend. The central theme is emergence – processes by which more complex systems arise from simpler systems, often unpredictably. This is the opposite of reductionism where any phenomenon can be explained by understanding the parts of that system. For example, orderly arrangement of molecules can appear simultaneously. Such emergent phenomena are common in everyday experience and sometimes require an energy input. Life on earth arose 46 million years ago. The question is posed of where organic compounds came from to start life and why is life chiral (handed) where mixtures of molecules rotate to the left or right. Even though God said (Genesis 1:20), 'Let the waters bring forth swarms of living creatures', such processes in life must be subject to the laws of chemistry and physics. Life may be organised as a chemical consequence given the appropriate environment and time, ideas which should be able to be tested by experiment. One of the consequences of interaction among carbon-based molecules is to assemble life's membranes, proteins, and genetic molecules on rocks and minerals. Many of Hazen's ideas are stimulated by discussion with Gunter Wachtershauser who was a chemist and patent lawyer and a friend of the philosopher Karl Popper who said that theories to be theories at all in the scientific sense must make testable predictions that have the potential to be proved false by empirical test. If predictions are precise, the more believable they are to scrutiny. If the 'primordial soup' concept of life is rejected, there are three other plausible assumptions:

1. The first life form made its own molecules as autotrophs, building its own molecular building blocks from scratch.
2. The first life form relied on the chemical energy of minerals, not the sun, and these are relatively simple like modern cellular processes.
3. Metabolism came first. This does not require encapsulation and membranes and excludes life beginning with a self-replicating model like RNA.

The ideas are amplified by the additional assumption of biological continuity in detailed chain reactions. The central chemical idea is that iron and nickel sulphides served as the template, catalyst, and energy source for biosynthesis. However, the ideas are controversial because nothing is proven. The primary goal is carbon fixation in prebiotic synthesis, and life must lead to bigger molecules. Minerals are likely to be very important as they are in all cell functions. Prebiotic synthesis gives a 50:50 mixture of chiral molecules. Living cells choose right-handed sugars over left, and left-handed amino acids over right. This 'homochirality' has never been explained. Such chiral chemistry is like the formation of a crystal and minerals often display beautiful crystal faces, which might have provided the ideal template for the assembly of life's molecules. The citric acid or TCA biochemical pathway was discovered by Hans Krebs and is used by all aerobic organisms to release stored energy through oxidation of a substance acetate derived from carbohydrates, fats, and proteins into carbon dioxide. By contrast, the reverse citric acid cycle is used by some bacteria to produce carbon compounds from carbon dioxide. It is Hazen's view that this may have been the engine for life's first metabolic process. Interestingly, on my first day, I arrived to teach microbiology in Oxford in 1980. I had lunch in St. John's College and was discussing my ideas on biogenesis of catabolism of gaseous hydrocarbons with one of my new colleagues across the table. He suggested that I should explore the citric acid cycles as the simplest explanation. His ideas made sense to me, and it was not until I asked his name that I found he was Hans Krebs!

In summary, Hazen provides three scenarios for the origin of life:

1. Life began with metabolism, and genetic molecules were incorporated later by the reverse citric acid cycle. It emerged from the chemical coating on rocks. While only partly tested, it could be the model to beat after full testing.
2. Life began with self-replicating genetic molecules, and metabolism was incorporated later. Organic molecules in the prebiotic soup, perhaps aided by clays or some other template, self-organised into information-rich polymers, and these eventually self-replicated.
3. Life began as a cooperative chemical phenomenon arising between metabolism and genetics, essentially a dual origin, probably occurring in early cellular life. Such symbiosis of metabolic cycle and an RNA-like genetic polymer is an attractive scenario.

The Miller-Urey investigations are discussed by Michael Marshall in his book published in 2020 *The Genesis Quest. The Geniuses and Eccentrics on a Journey to Uncover Life on Earth*. The distinctive approach of Marshall is that he provides detail on the character of the people involved in all the studies he considers. For example, he points out that Carl Sagan, who is discussed in Chapter 2, had his early career with Cyril Ponnamperuma at the NASA Ames Research Centre in California. At the age of 30, he was being divorced by his first wife, microbiologist Lynn Margulis because he was over-focussed on his career and did not help raise their two children, leaving her own career in limbo. Lynn went on to become one of the most influential biologists of the twentieth century. She collaborated with Carl Woese on the concept of the Last Universal Common Ancestor, and particularly on the distinction between prokaryotic and eukaryotic cells which is discussed in Chapter 1. They discussed the split between archaea and bacteria 3.4 billion years ago based on genetic evidence. The eukaryotes arose much later in a process where a bacterium wound up inside another cell, perhaps an archaean. Interestingly, Lynn Margulis wrote a dust jacket support for Hazen's book above. Such insights into the lives of leading scientists I have always found to be interesting, and it was one of the factors that stimulated me to follow a career in science. As a postgraduate student, I joined the research groups at Queen Elizabeth (now King's) College London of Clive Bird in organic chemistry and John Pirt where the focus was microbial growth. The other architect of the theory of microbial growth was Jacques Monod who had done his own PhD on the topic, showing the independence of growth rate and growth yield in submerged bacterial culture but went on to get the Nobel Prize for Physiology and Medicine in 1965 for his work showing that messenger RNA is a key factor in cell function. He became Director of the Institute Pasteur in Paris in 1971 but tragically died in 1977 aged 66. Monod also addressed the origin of life in his 1970 book *Chance and Necessity*. He argued that the origin of life on earth as such was extremely unlikely. He aligned with existentialist philosophers like Jean-Paul Sartre and Albert Camus who argued that life needs the moral compass of a God. He argued that evolution of new species is ultimately driven by random changes in genes and evolution was pure chance. Not surprisingly, this view has been heavily criticised. The opposite view is that was predestined. One of the leaders of the alternative view was the Belgian cell biologist Christian de Duve. He argued that life is a cosmic imperative and not arisen by chance in his book *Vital Dust*. The reality is that the truth is somewhere between the Monod and de Duve views. Vitalism assumes that there is something about living matter that makes it different from non-living matter. In the Book of Genesis (1:20), God said, 'Let the waters bring forth swarms of living creatures', but such processes must be subject to the laws of chemistry and physics unless they are miracles, but most likely the words are metaphorical to communicate with people of the time. He gave us dominium over creation and freewill and so many of the world's problems arise from the latter. In Genesis (2:7), it is stated, 'And the Lord God formed man of the dust of the ground and breathed into his nostrils the breath of life; and man became living being'. We have found in the pandemic that a principal action of COVID-19 is to deny the breath of life. Life is special and vitalism is a view of it. However, there has been no life force ever identified, which makes vitalism intuitive, and there have been many critics. Within the discussions, the issue of spontaneous generation has also been analysed. The theologians St. Augustine and St. Thomas Aquinas supported it but by the seventeenth century, the dogma had shifted, and the Church rejected it. The French naturalist Felix-Archimede Pouchet did an experiment in 1858 showing that hay infused water under mercury in sterile water under mercury went mouldy, suggesting this was spontaneous generation. The French Academy of Sciences was unsympathetic to the claims and launched a competition to disprove it. The competition was won by Louis Pasteur who showed that Pouchet had not been careful enough and showed that the layer of mercury was contaminated by microorganisms. This approach became vital in the discipline of microbiology which developed in the twentieth century where one of the first things we learnt was how to practically keep systems clean and sterile to sensible experiments. With the disproof of spontaneous generation as a route to the origin of life, other routes were considered and the great naturalist Charles Darwin published *On the Origin of Species* in 1859, but the reality is that this did not discuss the origin of life as such; it was instead focussed on evolution. It did not stop him coming into major conflict with Christians who thought he was trying to denigrate God as the creator of life. The book by Marshall uses the NASA definition that 'Life is a system capable of Darwinian evolution'. But he also questions if life is a concept that we are imposing on reality, not something that can be objectively defined. Even though we have the potential to self-destruct, as will be discussed in the next chapter, cosmologists can provide many reasons why in the long term the planet as we know it today will no longer support life. This pessimistic Doomsday scenario does not help us to think constructively about the earth as our cradle, our home, and our parent. There is nowhere else realistically for us to go and when society threatens to tear us apart; our living planet can bind us together.

To contemplate the origin of life, there is specific discipline that holds all the cards. We have already seen that philosophers, theologians, and scientists have all expressed their views over the centuries but there has been little comment so far on the role of historians. A notable exception to this is David Christian, Distinguished Professor of History at Macquarie University in Australia, produced *Origin Story. A Big History of Everything* in 2018. This book written in elegant and understandable prose covers all the ground I have covered thus far. It is built on a series of nine thresholds (timelines) of approximate dates with events taking place in them:

Threshold 1: (13.8 billion years ago) Big Bang and origin of universe.
Threshold 2: (13.2 billion years ago) The first stars begin to glow.
Threshold 3: (Threshold 2 to present) New elements formed in dying large stars.
Threshold 4: (4.5 billion years ago) Our sun and solar system form.
Threshold 5: (3.8 billion to million years ago) Earliest life on earth to emergence of *Homo erectus*.
Threshold 6: (200,000 years ago) First evidence of our species *Homo sapiens*.
Threshold 7: (10,000 to 500 years ago) End of last ice age, beginning of Holocene, earliest signs of farming through to world zones begin to be linked together.

Threshold 8: (200 to 50 years ago) Fossil fuel revolution beginning through to the great acceleration with humans landing on moon.

Threshold 9: The future.

The emergence of bacterial life forms in threshold 3 also depended on food sources. Indeed, capitalising on the pioneering work on microbial growth by Jacques Monod referred to above, the seminal contribution of my own PhD supervisor John Pirt was to describe the concept of maintenance energy which was necessary to keep the bacterial cell alive. This can be very low and indeed some cells adapt starvation by using their own internal energy reserves which can sometimes be aided by changing cell structures and forming spores. However, there will always be a tipping point where death will ultimately happen. Within these timelines, the earliest signs of farming at the beginning of threshold 7 took about another 5000 years for agrarian civilisations. This was of course the main route to sustaining life on the planet. This is discussed at length in Christian's book but will also be discussed in the next chapter of this book. His final threshold 8 before discussing The Future is the Anthropocene. This is not a recognised period like the epochs discussed earlier but represents modern times starting about 200 years ago. It is the current geological age, viewed as the period during which human activity has been the dominant influence on climate and the environment. Gaia Vince wrote a book in 2014 *Adventures in the Anthropocene. A Journey to the Heart of the Planet We Made*. She quit her job at the journal *Nature* to travel the world to explain these influences. She considers atmosphere, mountains, rivers, farmlands, oceans, deserts, savannahs, forests, rocks, and cities. That provides the platform to move to the analysis of how we have managed life in modern times, what we are doing today to protect it, and what we need to do to protect it for future generations.

4 Science and the Health of the Planet

Man has lost the capacity to foresee and to forestall. He will end by destroying the earth.

Albert Schweitzer 1875–1965

The Earth will not continue to offer its harvest, except with faithful stewardship.

We cannot say we love the land and then take steps to destroy it for use by future generations.

Pope John Paul II 1920–2005

I have discussed in the previous chapters how the planet and its associated life might have originated. Life in all its variety is amazing and well worth protecting. Even though the warning above giving by the Nobel Peace Prize laureate Albert Schweitzer, who was a polymath with skills which included medicine, music, and theology, may sound ominous, it is amazing how little attention has been paid to it. The message from Pope John Paul II restated the same message in essence more recently but gives hope by suggesting stewardship as the route to avoid destruction. As a student I was inspired by the book published in 1992 by Rachel Carson *Silent Spring* which focussed on the danger of pesticides, particularly DDT, being applied in the environment and entering the food chain. She was a marine biologist, but to put over her points she used emotive prose; chapter titles in the book included 'Elixirs of Death', 'And No Birds Sing', 'Rivers of Death', and 'The Human Price'. Most of her arguments were sound and fortunately the use of DDT was eventually banned under the influence of regulators such as the United States Environmental Protection Agency, which was established in 1970. Ironically in his America First campaign, President Trump said that he would close the EPA to protect the nation's economy! I guess today that we might term Rachel Carson an activist in a very positive light. As an untrained person, Erin Brockovich in California, the subject of a film produced in 2000, understood that hexavalent chromium was a potent toxicant to which people were being exposed, yet the manufacturers were taking little action to prevent human exposure. She got a job in a law firm to successfully challenge them and eventually qualified as a lawyer. Clearly, there is a massive role for regulators and legal challenge in protecting the environment.

My first job was at the Agricultural and Food Research Council Letcombe Laboratory in Oxfordshire, which was moving from assessing the impact of environmental radioactivity on crops to researching the impact of minimal cultivation on crop productivity in wet anaerobic soils. The environmental radioactivity arose from the accident at the Windscale nuclear power plant, and the fear was that the

DOI: 10.1201/9781003304845-4

radioactive fallout could enter the food chain. Even bigger problems arose subsequently at Chernobyl and showed the fragility of life to man-made events, although, in recent years, nature does seem to be some recovery or 'bouncing back' there. Direct drilling techniques could potentially reduce energy and fertiliser inputs to agriculture and reduce labour provided yields which were similar as those achieved to conventional tillage agriculture using the plough. One of the complications was that more herbicide was necessary to control weeds; with weeds at the bottom of the food chain, they can be important for pollinators and herbivores. Generally, in the UK, the herbicide of choice was paraquat, manufactured by ICI, but there was also the arrival of glyphosate which had been developed by Monsanto in the USA and was especially effective by being translocated to the roots and prevent weed re-emergence. My original task at Letcombe as the first microbiologist on staff was to identify the microbial processes that might reduce crops yields in the wet soils. The plant physiologists identified ethylene, which is a plant growth regulator, as the key factor reducing plant growth and I was able to show in a paper to *Nature* that this was generated by the fungus *Mucor hiemalis* growing on straw using the amino acid methionine as the substrate. Unfortunately, shortly after Alan Smith in Australia wrote a follow-on paper to *Nature* in which he said that anaerobic bacteria were the cause, and the gas was fungistatic. A follow-on from me in *Nature* showed that his experiments were flawed, and my original interpretation stood. The point of this story is to show the nature of scientific investigation and that even after peer review of papers in high-quality journals, interpretations of data can be challenged, and counter challenged. This applies equally well to the physical and chemical studies described in the previous two chapters as does to experiments in the natural environment and the infectious diseases that will be described in the next chapter.

Having resolved the ethylene story, I was approached with funding, first from Monsanto and then from ICI, to investigate the poor establishment observed after use by farmers of their herbicides. We showed that the adverse effect was not due to residual herbicide but due to the pathogen *Fusarium oxysporum* colonising the weed plant residues and infecting the establishing cereal crops. An important feature of glyphosate has been after many years of use and investigation; it has no toxicity to non-target organisms, including man. I found both Monsanto and ICI very ethical companies to work with. Similar approaches on minimal cultivation were being tested by the United States Department of Agriculture in the Pacific Northwest and I went to work with them at Washington State University. They were also investigating the appropriateness of organic farming. The Palouse sandy loam soils of the Pacific Northwest are very young in terms of cultivation with the area only being used for agriculture in the early twentieth century with the arrival of the wagon trains. Indeed, it was fascinating to meet some of the first settlers when I arrived in 1982. I was particularly impressed with their ingenuity in farming, and they seemed to get very good results from organic methods by attention to minute details in farming methods. As a result, they showed that good crop yields could be achieved with little or no input of fertilisers. This attracted great criticism from the Council for the Advancement of Scientific Technology, which is in fact a trade organisation supporting the fertiliser industry who felt threatened by the approach. Although it can be argued that the results in the Pacific Northwest could be influenced by the soils being so young and therefore rich in nitrogen, the results should be considered as we move to attempt lower-input farming systems.

Another factor which needs to be considered is crop rotation, a common feature of organic farming systems, as this can improve greatly the cycling of nutrients. Air travel has been a great technological innovation in the Anthropocene, but it also poses great threats with its emissions and a major contributor to climate change. Interestingly, despite the achievement of the space passenger launch by Richard Branson in July 2021, to be followed by others, many young people have been unenthusiastic and expressed concern that the emissions created are so damaging to the environment. Even the Astronomer Royal, Martin Rees, has questioned the cost with limited scientific benefit of the Space Station which has been flying for many years. I will come back to carbon emissions later in this chapter.

On my return from the USA, I was attracted by on offer by the Agricultural and Food Council (subsequently Biotechnology and Biological Sciences Research Council) to become Head of Department at Horticulture Research International in Littlehampton where research into biological control of pests and diseases had been pioneered and could reduce chemical input to the environment. This would become a major opportunity to reduce the input of chemicals into the environment. This will be covered in the next chapter.

To protect the planet, the only sensible approach is to take a holistic view and to take an interdisciplinary approach. One of the early advocates of such an approach has been James Lovelock in his 1979 book *Gaia*. Lovelock suggests that the earth is a living entity and functions as a single organism and that it can only be sustained by fostering all elements that contribute to that life. Lovelock described the complex entity of the earth's biosphere in relation to the atmosphere, oceans, and the soil. The totality of this constitutes a feedback or cybernetic system which seeks an optimal physical and chemical life on the planet. By maintaining relatively constant conditions with active control, the term 'homeostasis' can be applied to it. Many scientists criticised the approach of Lovelock as being soft. Many aspects of his commentary come from first-hand experience in working at NASA and subsequently developing the flame ionisation detector for use in gas chromatography to better study pollutants in the atmosphere and for which, along with his work formulating the *Gaia* Hypothesis, he became a Fellow of the Royal Society, a Commander of the Order of the British Empire, and a Companion of Honour. It is important that people writing in this arena come from a position of scientific strength, which likely means they will have an emphasis on their own expertise in providing analysis. Inevitably, the opportunity of the hard science approach is that quantification can usually be presented to substantiate the ideas expressed. An important approach is life cycle assessment (LCA), first formulated by Harold Smith at the World Energy Conference in 1963. It started to gain importance in the later part of the twentieth century but has only really attained prominence in this century. It is now the subject of standards set by the International Organisation of Standards. It provides methodology for assessing all stages of the life cycle of a commercial product, process, or service, through to its end of life, or cradle to grave. It can equally well be applied to health as well environmental processes such as ozone depletion and eutrophication. To become a Chartered Environmentalist in the UK, for which I was privileged to be an assessor,

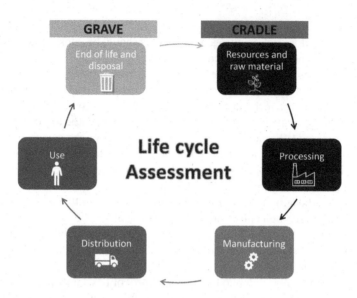

FIGURE 4.1   Life cycle assessment (LCA) from cradle to grave.

it is essential that candidates are fully familiar with LCA (Figure 4.1). It might be argued that this is a quantitative approach to analysing *Gaia*.

Clearly, the defence of life on the planet has an impact on politics but religious ministers must not engage on party politics, and they should instead engage on issues of life itself as we shall see in the final chapter. One of the most important contributions from a minister of religion on the issues of the science and health of the planet is the Encyclical letter by Pope Francis (2015) *Laudito Si'. On Care for Our Common Home.* This is an in-depth analysis of the health of the planet, very complementary to Gaia, but updated to cover issues such as climate change in a good depth. Pope Francis took his name from St. Francis of Assisi and indicates like St Francis that Mother Earth sustains and governs us but now cries out for help because of the harm we have inflicted on her. Inevitably, there is a gospel aspect about the Encyclical, mainly in Chapter 2, but largely it covers the environmental problems in an open and insightful manner. I do not know how widely it has been read but the title might be unappealing to some. He terms 'rapidification' as the continued acceleration of changes affecting humanity and the planet, coupled with an intensified pace of life and work. The Amazon and Congo basins are among the most biodiverse lungs of the planet. Yet we have often moved to the destruction of virgin forest with plantations of trees, often monocultures, the impacts of which is rarely analysed. In Scotland, with the post-World War II zeal to produce tree biomass quickly irrespective of how valuable it was, the destruction of soil structure on hillsides and loss of biodiversity resulted in the flow country saga. This was largely a consequence of planting monocultures of Sitka Spruce which are native to the Pacific Northwest. Even when I joined the Forestry Commission as CEO of the Research Agency in 2003, litigations from the Royal Society for the Protection of Birds were still live. I immediately supported a return to more mixed evergreen/deciduous stands along with a reduction in clear felling and towards natural regeneration. Pope Francis pays great attention to the welfare of poor people, and this is particularly true in forest communities. A total of 1.2 billion people, or a fifth of the World's population, depend on forests for their livelihood. As a member of the board of the European Forest Institute from 2016 to 2012, I was pleased to be involved in the creation by the European Union of the FLEGT (Forest Law Enforcement, Governance and Trade) Programme to combat illegal logging. Approximately 15%–30% of global forest production (50%–90% in tropical countries) is illegally logged, depressing timber prices by 16%. The primary victims of this are the indigenous people of the forests and it is those that need to be supported by international intervention. The only effective way to monitor this is with satellites (Figure 4.2), but in a paper to *Nature* in 2013, we argued

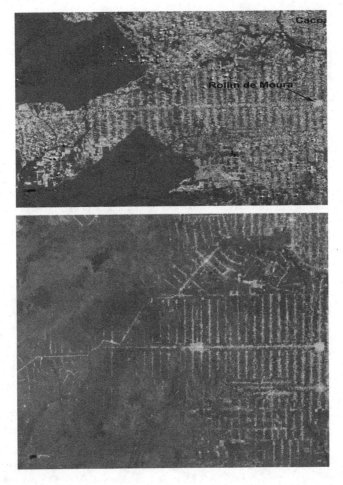

FIGURE 4.2 Deforestation in Rondônia, Brazilian Amazonia. The lower picture was taken in 1986 with the LANDSAT satellite system (30 m resolution) and shows mainly red (dark) colour from the tree cover. The upper picture taken at the same site in 2011 with DMC-2 (22 m resolution) shows extensive fishbone deforestation in blue (light) colour. DMC-2 images with permission of Airbus.

that there needs to be more international consensus of the monitoring, reporting, and verification deployed. One of the lead agencies globally in making these assessments is the Brazilian Space Agency (INPE) where we have collaborated from the UK (Figure 4.3). This is ever more important today as very high-resolution satellite imagery is available with resolutions down to 0.3 m (Figure 4.4) against the 22 m resolution which had been common. The higher resolution can detect individual trees

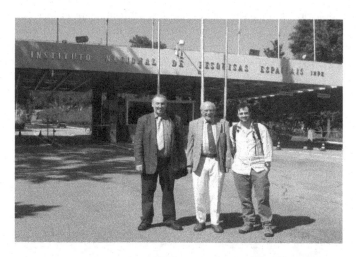

FIGURE 4.3   Visit to INPE (Brazilian Space Agency) with colleague Steve Morse (left) and our research student Mercio Cerbaro. Brazil has been a leader in earth observation globally but it remains to be seen if this will continue with President Bolsonaro a reduction of the budget of the ministry of science, technology and innovation (MCTI) of over 90% in late 2021, and there has been a cut in the INPE budget of 70% over the past 7 years.

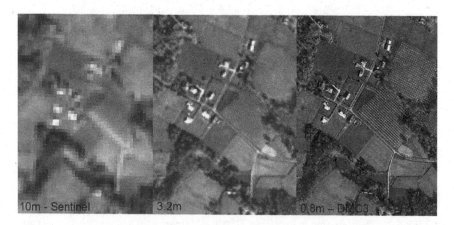

FIGURE 4.4   High resolution satellite imagery with Sentinel, 3.2m multispectral DMC-3 and 80cm hyperspectral DMC-3 satellite constellations. Multispectral images have 3-10 bands whereas hyperspectral have hundreds or thousands very narrow bands. Sentinel image with permission of the European Space Agency and DMC-3 images with permission of 21AT Asia.

and therefore capture the chain-saw loggers felling individual trees. Of course, care must be taken in the prosecution of such cases when detected because some native people are only felling of occasional trees to sustain the livelihood of their families. Pope Francis indicates that anthropocentrism, where mankind comes first rather than animals or God, is at the heart of what we do and there needs to be readjustment. Too much emphasis at times is devoted to a technocracy. What is needed is an integral ecological approach to life, involving environmental, economic, social, and cultural approaches.

In the UK, we have been lucky that the Royal Family have taken a keen interest in the preservation of the national and global environment. The speeches and writings from 1961 to 1987 of HRH Prince Philip (died 2021), Duke of Edinburgh, have been documented in his book published in 1988 *Down to Earth*. He became one of the world's leading conservationists and President of the World Wildlife Fund. Prince Philip was frequently outspoken, but this is necessary if impact is to be made. His considerations cover the exploitation of the natural system, the population factor, and the victims. He ends up with the moral imperative and considers the Declarations on Nature by the Hindu, Christian, Buddhist, Muslim, and Jewish faiths. There is remarkable consistency between the faiths. HRH the Prince of Wales, with Tony Juniper and Ian Skelly in *Harmony. A New Way of Looking at the World* published in 2010 develops further his father's views on considering what we have lost in the modern world and what is needed to meet the modern challenges, including those in the built environment, engineering, medicine, and farming. His philosophy on fields such architecture, the inner cities, education, religion, health, and farming are explained for the first time. Part of that is a result of that is reflected in the list of around 400 organisations of which he is President or Patron. My personal contact with his activities was the Rainforest Project in 2007, which was focussed on the tropics where he pragmatically ceded the lead role to Norway and merged his activity into his International Sustainability Unit. He points out that we are at an historic moment – because we face a future where there is a real prospect that if we fail the earth, we fail humanity. It is great to have royal support for sustainability and we should all be able to play our part, however small, in delivery. Sadly, this has often not been the case, especially at a high level. For example, the felling and burning of rainforest in the Amazonia to make way for farming and commercial activities has been strongly supported by the Brazilian President Bolsonaro, sometimes with implicit support from President Trump. This is on a great scale with massive global impacts.

On a small scale, but with massive local impact and the potential to roll out more widely, Isabella Tree produced her book *Wilding. The Return to Nature of a British Farm* in 2018. It is based on her work at the Knepp Castle Estate in West Sussex. Until these 3500 acres were a typically unprofitable farm based on monoculture; the land was polluted and degraded. She and her husband Charles Burrell had struggled for 17 years to make it profitable but failed. Then she had the idea of letting it grow wild with minimal human intervention. Herds of free-roaming animals stimulate new habitats, and the biodiversity has escalated. There are rare species such as turtle doves, peregrine falcons, and purple emperor butterflies now breeding. With free public access, I was highly impressed and stimulated by the environment on a recent visit. Visitors were made welcome and there is a farm shop to buy meat from their animals and a great campsite. They are essentially providing an ecosystem service. This can only be truly effective if the Government develops the concept of payments for ecosystem services (PES) through various initiatives. For example, there is great potential to increase biodiversity by stimulating the planting of hedgerows, which can also be a source of natural predators of pests and diseases, instead of destroying them which was a characteristic of monoculture food production. When I was CEO of the Forestry Commission Research Agency, we tried to open the land as the largest land holding in the UK to public access by providing more quality cycle tracks and footpaths. To study this and with EU grants, we were able to show that this provided health benefits to the people using the forests and land, especially to improve well-being. Some analysts showed that this had potentially a higher value than that of the timber itself. I held meetings with the Chief Medical Officers in each of the devolved UK countries who saw the enormous potential to improve health and well-being. At that time, the concept of PES was in its infancy but today this should be reconsidered. Essentially, the land provides a green gymnasium for people to improve their lives, provided we can support access to the areas, especially by those living in deprived areas of inner cities. There is also the potential for coniferous trees to exert direct pharmacological effects by the release of terpenes. Though cause and effect has not been proven, some surgeons in Germany found that patients had improved recovery from surgery by moving sanitoria from cities to country districts surrounded by trees. Traditionally, sanitoria were built in rural or coastal districts for surgery and recovery from diseases like tuberculosis. By contrast, a city like London had one of the highest infection rates. In the current COVID-19 pandemic, cities, especially in the North of England, also seem to have fared worst but that is large part is probably due to closer contact of individuals especially where housing is more cramped. Nevertheless, poor air quality in cities is likely linked to a variety of poor health conditions. Experience in the creation of the Central Scotland Forest on the site of former open-cast mines and encouraging people from socially deprived backgrounds to go for short walks has been of value.

One of the greatest concerns for the health of the planet in modern times has been gaseous emissions, which, amongst other things, cause climate change. In my opinion, one of the most important contributors to that theory was Roger Revelle. Most of his early research was at the Scripps Institute of Oceanography (SIO) in La Jolla, San Diego. I was privileged to visit SIO as Vice-Chair of the Blasker Award Committee of the San Diego Community Foundation in 1999, of which Rita Colwell was Chair. I met Revelle's collaborator, Charles Keeling, who provided me with a copy of the book by Judith and Neil Morgan *Roger: A Biography of Roger Revelle*, written in 1996, 5 years after his death. He collected gaseous samples every day to measure CO_2 concentrations at multiple locations round the world, over many years. He had as his main base Mauna Loa, a massive volcanic mountain on the big island of Hawaii which was untainted by local industrial emissions. His experiments were the first hard evidence that global CO_2 levels were rising. Revelle left SIO for Harvard in 1963, before returning to San Diego in 1976. While at Harvard, he taught Al Gore who was to become Vice-President of the United States between 1993 and 2001. Gore made a massive positive impact on US Environment Policy and during his tenure Rita Colwell became the first biologist and first woman to become Director of the National Science Foundation, a post she held from 1998 to 2004. Gore stood for election as President in 2000 but lost to George W. Bush narrowly after a very close and controversial recount in Florida. That triggered a reversal in US Climate Change Policy. It took until 2009 when Barack Obama was elected President to re-establish the positive approach to US Climate Policy, even though many industrialists were opposed with self-interest at heart. Just before Obama took office, I was privileged, as a Board Member of the OECD Programme for Biological Sustainability, to read his constructive plans communicated to OECD for climate action. Despite his challenges of a minority in the US Senate, he signed up to the important Paris Agreement of COP 21 in Paris in December 2015, where Pope Francis was also present to support the actions. Ironically, this was to no avail because during the Presidency of Donald Trump from 2017 to 2021, the US withdrew from the agreement. The turbulent presidency led to Trump being impeached for pressurising Ukraine to investigate his political rival Joe Biden in December 2019. I was fortunate to attend the hearings in the House of Representatives, sitting behind the former US Ambassador to the Ukraine, Marie Yovanovitch, while she testified that she was a victim of disinformation tactics, but who Trump recalled from her post. Fortunately, many important US states resisted Trump's actions on climate change so that when Joe Biden assumed the Presidency in 2022, he reaffirmed US support for the Paris Agreement. Some of the conclusions from the COP 26 Meeting in Glasgow in November 2022 are covered in the final chapter. In advance of the meeting, BBC screened a television 'Climategate' drama *The Trick* which described the excellent work of Phil Jones at the University of East Anglia Climatic Research Unit in which he was wrongly accused of scientific fraud by rigging data to exaggerate global warming by deniers hacking into his e-mails. This resulted in death threats on him, possibly in part initiated by vested commercial interests in the USA ahead of the 2009 COP 15 meeting in Copenhagen. Fortunately, he was subsequently exonerated by a parliamentary enquiry. He does, however, feel that the scandal was a 'David Kelly moment' like the 'sexed up' dossier of weapons of mass destruction described in Chapter 1. Clearly, the US engagement in Glasgow, with attendance by Joe Biden and John Kerry, was critical to make global reductions in emissions, but the challenge was to attempt to persuade large countries like China, who have steadily increased their emissions, to engage in some form even though as the largest producer of coal adjustment will be difficult. The US Presidential Election in 2000 could have changed Climate Change Policy had Al Gore been elected. Similarly, in the 2016 election, had Hilary Clinton been elected, there would have been a different approach to the environment. Ironically just before that election, I had a personal e-mail from Hilary Clinton as Governor of New York State congratulating Gary Harman of Cornell University and myself on forming a joint venture company between Cornell and Surrey Universities, Phytobials LLC, aimed at producing microbial inoculants for plants to reduce environmental load which will be discussed in the next chapter. The importance and impact of such political interventions on science will be discussed in the final chapter.

Al Gore continued to have a massive impact on US and global climate change policies. His book published in 2006 *An Inconvenient Truth. The Planet Emergency of Global Warming and What We Can Do about It* was also released as a major motion picture. This was followed with another book published in 2009 *Our Choice*.

A Plan to Solve the Climate Crisis to assess progress and provide actions. Gore starts the book by pointing out that greenhouse gases which are responsible for global warming are not just CO_2. Also important are methane and nitrous oxide which are on a unit basis more active than CO_2, although far less in volume, and they arise from industry, agriculture, and burning of forests. He then has a chapter on his scientific hero, Roger Revelle! The book is written very clearly describing the evidence for climate change, with excellent pictures and diagrams but also with many key 'punch' lines. For example:

- Almost all mountain glaciers in the world are now melting, many of them quite rapidly.
- In 2004, the record for tornadoes in the United States was broken.
- The insurance industry feels the economic impact of global warming which over the past three decades has seen a 15-fold increase in payments to victims of extreme weather.
- Drunken' trees in Alaska put their roots deep into the frozen tundra and now as it melts, they lose their anchor and sway in all directions.
- The link between global warming and large-scale bleaching of corals in universally accepted.
- Some 30 so-called new diseases have emerged over the past 30 years and some old diseases are surging again.
- Many residents of low-lying Pacific Islands have already had to evacuate because of rising seas.
- The maps of the world will have to be redrawn (quoting Sir David King, UK Scientific Advisor).
- The way we treat forests is a political issue.
- The contributions to global warming are the USA (30.3%), Europe (27.7%), Russia (13.7%), and Southeast Asia, India, and China (12.2%).
- Of the peer-reviewed scientific articles (928) on climate change published in previous 10 years before the book none had any doubt as to cause of global warming. By contrast, in the 636 popular press articles in the previous 14 years, 53% doubted the cause of global warming.

In the second of Gore's books, he points out some of the solutions and problems such as:

- Quoting Thomas Edison 'I'd put my money on the sun and solar energy. What a source of power!'
- In the past 2 years, wind power has been the greatest source of increased electricity-generation in the United States.
- Quoting Stephen Chu, US Secretary of Energy 'The amount of geothermal energy potentially available is effectively unlimited'.
- Biomass energy is one of the most promising ways to reduce significant amounts of CO_2 from the burning of coal and natural gas but producing first-generation ethanol from corn is a mistake.

- The idea of a 'capture ready' coal plant is yet unproven and unlikely to be fruitful.
- Nuclear power, once expected to provide unlimited supplies of low-cost electricity, has been an energy source in crisis for the last 30 years.
- The CO_2 emissions from deforestation are second only to the burning of fossil fuels, to produce electricity and heat, as the largest source of global warming on the planet.
- Soil plays an active role in the earth's carbon cycle, storing an estimated three to four-and-a half times as much carbon as the earth's plant matter combined.
- Industrial agriculture now uses 10 calories of energy from fossil fuels to produce one calorie in food.
- The technologies necessary to build a super grid are all fully developed and available now.
- Global warming has often been described as the greatest market failure in history.
- The choice is awesome and potentially eternal. It is in the hands of the present generation.

Hopefully, we will move to accept and adopt more of Gore's recommendations as we try to safeguard the planet. Gore won the 2007 Nobel Peace Prize for his initiatives on climate change. The last bullet pony is particularly salutary and supports the action of the 15-year-old Norwegian Greta Thunberg in 2018 generating school strikes for climate. It is crucial that younger people are fully engaged with the need to tackle climate change. A group of young Catholics in the Ecological Conversion Group led by John Paul De Quay (aged 33) with the support of Bishops Richard Moth (Arundel and Brighton) and John Arnold (Salford) produced a valuable booklet *The Journey to 2030*. Imagery of the problems can be important, and I was impressed with an exhibit (www.felicityorourkegardendesign.com/rhs-global-impact-garden-extinction) at the Hampton Court Garden Festival in July 2021 by Felicity O'Rourke who trained in biochemistry and is a former airline pilot turned garden designer (Figure 4.5). The plane crash symbolises our own personal vulnerability to inspire individual choices to change. The garden consists of three elements.

- **Wheat**: represents man's attempt to dominate nature which ironically has resulted in mankind becoming a slave to modern agricultural methods.
- **The aircraft:** not only represents an arresting, in-your-face image which triggers all those raw emotions but represents our dominance of the world of science and technology. While aircraft contribute to CO_2 emissions, their contribution is relatively small compared with that of global shipping, for example. So, the aircraft is used to highlight our dominance of nature and the world and show that although we are the dominant species on earth, we are not superior, and we are certainly not immune to extinction. The aircraft acts as a portal to see beyond the present day to the third element of the garden, the primordial planting.

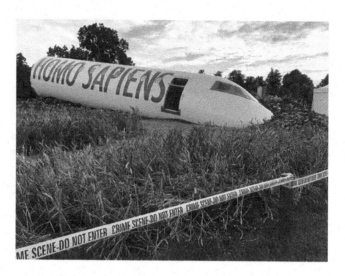

FIGURE 4.5   Extinction? (Felicity O'Rourke)

- **The primordial planting**: (on the far side of the fuselage) represents the
  lush, rich nature which existed long before our evolution on earth and represents those species which will survive us should a sixth mass extinction
  event result in the demise of humanity. Its presence here instils humility
  in the onlooker, reaffirming our own vulnerability and showcasing true
  survivors.

Gore had a large team of people working with him to produce his analyses. More
recently, Bill Gates with another large team produced an updated analysis in his
book published in 2020 *How to Avoid a Climate Crisis. The Solutions We Have and
the Breakthroughs We Need.* He starts by telling us that there are two numbers we
need to know about climate change. Fifty-one billion is how many tons of greenhouse gases the world typically adds to the atmosphere every year, zero is what we
need to aim for. Unsurprisingly from his background, his options are innovative and
commercially sound. He is also optimistic. His afterword chapter considers climate
change and COVID-19. His vast experience in supporting global health and farming
philanthropically has high relevance to the climate crisis and he has just three bullet
points

- We need international cooperation.
- We need to let science – actually, many different sciences – guide our efforts.
- Our solutions should meet the needs of people who are hardest hit.

These comments chine with the philosophy of people like Pope Francis which we
have already discussed in this chapter.

Gates particularly acknowledges the science and practical approach that was
taken by Sir David MacKay. He was appointed Professor of Physics at Cambridge
at the young age of 36 and in 2009 was appointed Chief Scientific Advisor to the

Department of Energy and Climate Change. I met him over dinner with Sir David King (UK Chief Scientific Adviser) at the Geological Society that year. He passed me a copy of the new book he had just written *Sustainable Energy – without the Hot Air*. It shows quantitatively how we can replace fossil fuels, ensure energy supply, and solve climate change. It is wide ranging and so relevant today. When he returned to Cambridge in 2014, he was made Regius Professor of Engineering but tragically he died of cancer in 2016, aged 48. In my opinion, his book should have been essential reading for attendees at COP 26 in Glasgow in 2021.

Gore and Gates are consistent on their views on the value of science. For example, Gore's comment above on producing ethanol from corn was a mistake, justified by the big increase in corn prices such that Midwest farmers could no longer afford corn to feed cattle potentially, compromising beef supply. This type of enigma is taken further in the book edited by John Love and John Bryant in 2017 *Biofuels and Bioenergy*. The book takes a very wide perspective, including the very important options of algae. That is an arena in which I have taken an interest, especially the massive mats of the red halo-tolerant alga *Duniella* which cover the coasts of Namibia. With the saline stress, over 85% of the cell mass is glycerol. If the alga is harvested, and the glycerol extracted, it could be burnt in modified diesel engines for the generation of power. However, this has not yet been exploited commercially. In the final chapter of the book on the ethical aspects of biofuels, the conclusion is made by Bryant and Hughes that 'they and Jim Lynch (in the previous chapter, Sustainability of Biofuels), emphasise that biofuel production *can* be a social and environmental good, but it will take deep wisdom and good governance to ensure that it is so'. It seems to me that ethics and LCA should be considered in all environmental analyses; I will return to this in Chapter 6.

In terms of mathematical analysis and prediction of scientific and environmental effects, it is important to distinguish linear and non-linear systems. Linear law, in which 'effect' is directly proportional to cause', is simply a straight line (Figure 4.6). However, most physical laws, such as Newton's inverse-square law of gravity, are not linear. Some simple non-linear problems can be solved with pencil and paper; it does not take long for a non-linear problem to become intractable, such as Newton's inverse-square law to compute the motion of three planets under the influence of gravitational forces, the feedback creating a Gordian Knot (an intricate problem, especially a problem insoluble in its own terms). In non-linear systems, the change in the output is not proportional to the change of the input and therefore the equations look more complicated. In the extreme of non-linear systems, stochastic dynamics are always random. However, when random states of disorder are governed by underlying patterns and laws, the system is said to be chaotic and governed by deterministic patterns and deterministic laws. The patterns formed, often in the shape of a butterfly, were first described by Edward Lorenz and are known as strange attractors. The book by James Gleick *Chaos. Making a New Science* is a great introduction to the subject. My first entry into investigating chaos was in analysing and finding the strange attractor pattern in the predator-prey interaction of protozoan amoebae grazing on bacteria in a stirred tank. However, by far, the most important analyses have been in predicting the weather. This has been described in the book by Ian Roulstone and John Norbury *Invisible in the Storm. The Role of Mathematics in Understanding*

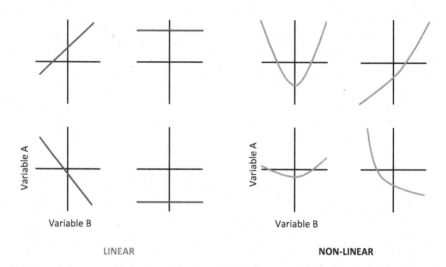

FIGURE 4.6 Linear and non-linear functions. The linear function has something to do with a line and can be a simple equation like $y = mx + b$. The non-linear function includes periodic (repeats its values at regular intervals), quasi-periodic (repeats its values at irregular intervals), sub-harmonic, and chaotic functions and includes differential equations. Non-linear functions include logarithmic and exponential systems such as $y = \log_{10}(x)$.

Weather. The importance of complex physical systems in deciphering chaotic climate was recognised by the award of the 2021 Nobel Prize in Physics to Syukuro Manabe (USA), Klaus Hasselman (Germany), and Giorgio Parisi (Italy). It is so important for such fundamental science to be translated into policy in attempts to combat climate change as well as using the concepts in cognate arenas. My interaction with Ian Roulstone has shown that forests can show non-linear behaviour as they reach a tipping point and die, which can be caused by environmental factors such as the weather, potentially being enhanced by climate change where trees cannot tolerate higher temperatures. The tipping point can also potentially be precipitated by pests and diseases. In that respect, diseases of animals and man might exhibit this non-linear behaviour. The current COVID-19 pandemic has been analysed extensively at the statistical level to produce models of infection and death, but few of the models have been non-linear, even chaotic. This must surely be worthy of further investigation in the attempt to describe the science and health of the planet mathematically. It should be recognised that systems can be stable against stressors in equilibrium theory.

Quantitative analysis should be at the heart of sustainability and biology should be the driver. An overview of this is provided by Stephen Morse in his book *Sustainability. A Biological Perspective.* Sustainability enhances the domains of environment, economy, and community (Figure 4.7). Critical sustainability is not effective if it does not meet economic goals nor if it does not allow for the well-being and development of communities. *De facto*, it is a highly interdisciplinary approach to life which is often not recognised by academic communities and referees of publications in the field. Having been an assessor for the award of Chartered

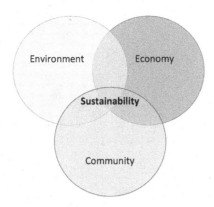

FIGURE 4.7 The interlocking circles of sustainability.

Environmentalist, I have been impressed by the rigour of evaluation for candidates in understanding of sustainability as a primary requirement, including the quantitative analysis of LCA. The book by Morse gives many examples of quantitative analysis in sustainability assessments, especially by using sustainability indicators and indices. In the analysis of fisheries, he again goes into the use of chaos theory and identification of strange attractors. He spent 10 years working in Nigeria on protecting the agricultural environment with a strong emphasis on protecting the life and well-being of communities, using funding by the Catholic Church, and, more recently, improving yam production which has been funded by the Gates Foundation. I have worked with him in recent years on the remote sensing analysis of deforestation in Amazonia and the protection indigenous communities. Most recently, we have been using satellite imagery to assess some of the 17 UN Sustainable Development Goals (SDGs) (Figure 4.8), including monitoring, reporting, and verification within environmental land management policy, and assessment of soil carbon which is critical in the full analysis of the carbon cycle.

One of the greatest challenges we face is food security, along with the problems created by climate change and water supply, all of which are closely inter-related. An article in the August 2021 issue of *National Geographic* magazine discusses food insecurity in the USA which is defined as a lack of consistent access to enough food for a healthy life and indicates that an estimated 45 million people fall into that category, exacerbated by the COVID-19 pandemic. Unemployment and poverty can be drivers, and this can place a particular burden on the homeless and communities of colour. This is almost certainly a global problem and many countries without access to less charities and community kitchens will be even harder hit.

At Surrey with my colleague Jhuma Sadhukhan, we have assessed the sustainability of food production systems with a particular focus on the waste generated and its potential for biorefining in a circular economy (Figure 4.9). Traditionally, products are promoted in a linear economy that ignores recoverable resources and creates negative social and environmental impacts. This could be avoided with sustainable diets, valorisation of unavoidable wastes in the food chain, valuing food in line the UN SDGs which could be 'Game Changers'. For a sustainable diet, comprehensive

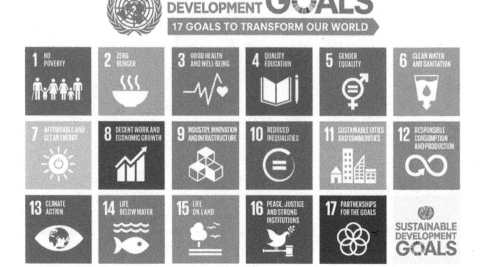

FIGURE 4.8   Sustainable Development Goals (SDGs).

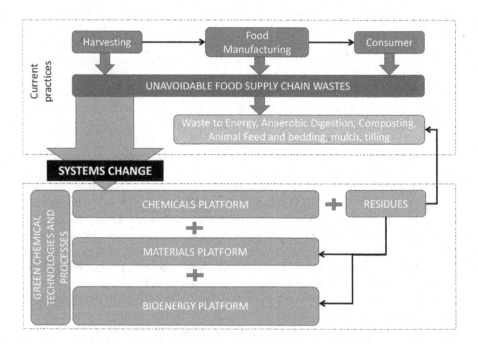

FIGURE 4.9 Systems change in unavoidable food waste biorefinery approach. (*Sustainability*, 2020, *12*, 1976. This is an open-access article distributed under the Creative Commons Attribution Licence which permits unrestricted use, distribution, and reproduction in any medium, provided the original work is properly cited.)

LCA is required by using global LCA datasets, and recommended daily servings are used rank food choices. All food groups from fresh fruits/vegetables, lentils/pulses, and grains to livestock need to be assessed, in relation to health and the environment. Likely emphasis is on a plant-based diet, especially plant-based sources of protein, with holistic systemic sustainability at the heart for the stability of the earth system. To avoid food chain wastes, economically feasible integrative innovative biorefinery systems are needed to provide functional and platform chemical productions, including nutraceuticals, or industrial symbiosis as well as energy in the form of fuel or combined heat and power. This quantitative circular economy approach to the protection of life on the planet should stimulate dietary change and provide real hope for the future.

It is useful to reflect how land is used globally (Figure 4.10), with useful land for agriculture and forestry being compromised by desertification, especially in a climate change scenario and where natural forests which are effective in capturing carbon dioxide are being cleared for agriculture. Land is a finite resource as is admirably expressed in the quotations at the start of this chapter. Economic analysis is critical if we are to protect the planet without compromising standards of living and thereby engaging the support of all society. The use of LCA is critical to achieve this

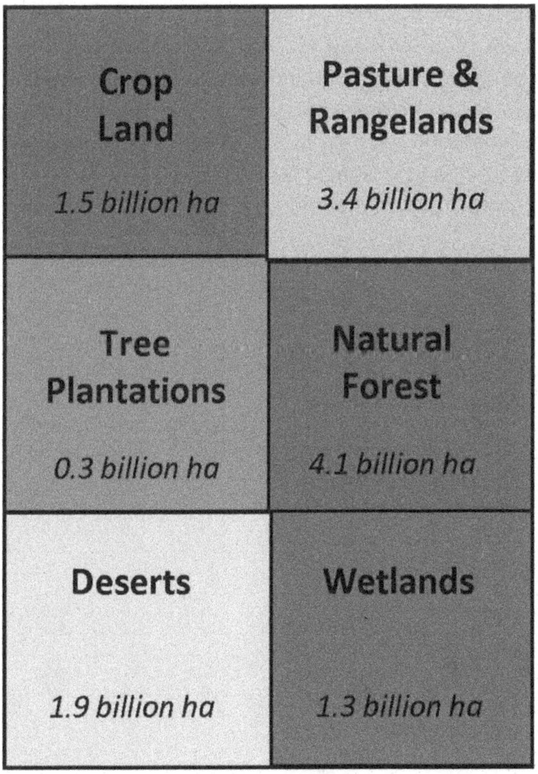

Crop Land 1.5 billion ha	Pasture & Rangelands 3.4 billion ha
Tree Plantations 0.3 billion ha	Natural Forest 4.1 billion ha
Deserts 1.9 billion ha	Wetlands 1.3 billion ha

FIGURE 4.10 Global land use.

and natural capital that is essential to sustain life on the planet must be part of the equation. Important in that respect is the concept of PES is built into the economic equations. For example, forests have timber production as their primary drive but the social and health benefits of people using forests for recreation can outweigh the timber value if managed appropriately, as can flood risk reduction and carbon capture to limit climate change. As one of the major global contributors to economic analysis, OECD has always considered carefully how much growth in the economy can be achieved sustainably. It was therefore stimulating when my colleague at Surrey Tim Jackson published his book in 2009 *Prosperity without Growth. Economics for a Finite Planet*. He has been invited to deliver the concepts of his new economics to a wide range of international bodies, including the UN General Assembly. Of particular concern is the use of the term gross domestic product as a measure of 'economic activity' in a nation or region. This term has been used for a century and is appealing to the world's poorest nations, but does it give a measure of true prosperity and address the billion people in the world who live on less than $1 per day? In a world of 6.7 billion people, 4 billion still live without basic entitlements. The Club of Rome's *Limits to Growth* published in the 1970s laid out the warnings but the idea of a nongrowing economy is an anathema to most economists in contrast to ecologists seeing a continually growing economy as an anathema. Post-war economic growth has largely been a story of unsustainable development and new blueprints such as those outlined in Jackson's book need appraisal urgently. We need to redefine prosperity, sort out the dilemma of growth and the myth of 'decoupling' in which production processes are reconfigured and good and services redesigned, such that economic output becomes less dependent on material throughput to attempt sustain resources. Currently, during pandemic, we are facing a shortage economy, involving issuers such as energy and food, and this must be managed for sustainability to be effective. Microbes are key drivers of sustainability.

5 Spread and Control of Microbes

Microbes are doing things we didn't even know they could 10 years ago.

Robert H. Jackson 1892–1954

It is obvious that human (and non-human) diseases are evolving with an unusual rapidity simply because our behaviour facilitate cross-fertilization of different strains of germs as never before, while an unending flow of new medicines (and pesticides) also present infectious organisms with rigorous, changing challenges to their survival.

William H. McNeil 1917–2016

The discovery of microbes as animalcules by Antonie van Leeuwenhoek was made possible with the development of the microscope as was discussed in Chapter 2. These rod or spherical (coccus) forms were bacteria of around 1 μm in size. It took much longer with the development of the powerful electron microscope by Ernst Ruska in 1931 to visualise viruses which are often only about one-tenth the size of bacteria and are not cells but packages of nucleic acids (RNA or DNA), surrounded by a protective coat called a capsid. Some larger viruses can be as big as bacteria but COVID-19, for example, is only about one-tenth of a micrometre. The science of microbiology developed with bacteria, along with cellular fungi and protozoa, in one stream, and viruses in another. In common, they all have nucleic acids which have only been characterised since James Watson and Francis Crick discovered the double helix structure of DNA in 1953. Medicine has usually been concerned with the microbes that cause disease, but some have beneficial effects such as those which aid digestion in the gut. Microbes in the environment can be harmful, such as those which cause plant diseases, or beneficial, such as those which improve plant nutrient cycling and those which break down pollutants. Most identification and early studies in the laboratory were with single species in pure culture, although viruses could only be grown with host animal or plant cells. This contrasts the real world where microbes associate with each other in microbial communities.

One of the major successes in the control of microbes was the discovery of antibiotics, firstly by Alexander Fleming in showing that the fungus *Penicillium notatum* from the air growing on an agar plate could control bacterial development. This led to the production of penicillin by fermentation by Ernst Chain in Rome and the clinical application by Howard Florey in Oxford, and the award of the Nobel Prize in Physiology or Medicine in 1945 to the three of them. In 1953, Selman Waksman having produced streptomycin from the soil bacterium *Streptomyces* to control tuberculosis (TB) was also awarded the Nobel Prize in Physiology or Medicine. His autobiography *My Life with Microbes* published in 1958 highlights the importance of soil

DOI: 10.1201/9781003304845-5

microorganisms in the search for antibiotics. These discoveries heralded a new wave of medicine where it was felt that antibiotics would cure most infectious diseases. What was not reckoned was that infectious agents would build up resistance to anti-biotics and that the pharmaceutical industry reduced its interest in developing new agents, largely because of cost. Even with the move to vaccines in treatment, there is still a need for antibiotics to be developed against a range of diseases.

Having studied microbiology at the postgraduate level in the laboratory, it struck me that there was a need to investigate microorganisms living in the environment, so in 1975 I became the first Convenor of the Society for General Microbiology (now the Microbiology Society) Ecology Group. This provided a forum for discussion nation-ally, linking to the International Microbial Ecology symposia started in 1977. With Nigel Poole, I edited a volume *Microbial Ecology. A Conceptual Approach* in 1979 for Blackwell, which had a follow-up with John Hobbie as my co-editor in 1988 *Micro-organisms in Action. Concepts and Applications in Microbial Ecology.* The latter introduced the topics of aerobiology, viral ecology, extreme environments, plasmids, and biological control. It was stimulating to work in Oxford with Robert Campbell of Blackwell Scientific Publications as the commissioning editor, in part because Robert May was writing his book on *Theoretical Ecology. Principles and Applications* and John Krebs was writing his book on *Behavioural Ecology. An Evolutionary Approach* at the same time, so that we could discuss parallels. It also encouraged me to produce my lectures at Oxford into another Blackwell book *Soil Biotechnology. Microbiological Factors in Crop Productivity* which defined a new discipline in 1983. Work with pure or even mixed cultures of microbes isolated from the environment (autecology) has value in understanding their physiological and bio-chemical behaviour, studying organisms in situ in a particular environment (synecol-ogy) leads to a fuller understanding of their dynamics. For example, in a paper to *Nature* by Eric Senior, Alan Bull, and Howard Slater in 1976, it was shown that using a mixed culture growing in a steady-state stirred reactor in the laboratory (a chemo-stat) that the herbicide Dalapon is degraded by a stable microbial community of seven members. One member, *Pseudomonas putida*, acquired the ability to grow on the herbicide through the evolution of a dehalogenase enzyme. In my own laboratory, in another paper to *Nature*, Duncan Veal and I showed that a cellulose-degrading fungus, *Trichoderma harzianum*, could co-operate with an anaerobic nitrogen-fixing bacterium *Clostridium butyricum*, in an aerobic atmosphere associated with the bac-terium *Enterobacter cloacae*. The latter produced polysaccharide gel for respiratory protection, allowing the aerobe and the anaerobe to function together. Such associa-tions almost certainly function in the natural environment. *T. harzianum* also hap-pens to function well to control plant diseases and has been used on a commercial scale, but again it likely functions most efficiently by producing associations with other microorganisms. John Whipps joined my laboratory at Letcombe (Oxfordshire) in 1977 and initially we produced an experimental model to investigate how micro-organisms got their energy to grow in soil from plant roots by using plant growth chambers as close to the natural environment as possible. The atmosphere was aer-ated but sealed and we introduced carbon dioxide labelled with the radioactive iso-tope carbon-14. As the plant photosynthesised, we could then track the fate of the photosynthate captured. We found that about 40% of the carbon captured was released by roots in what we termed rhizodeposition. Much of it was as polysaccharide gels which could be utilised by microorganisms and turned into microbial biomass, which, in turn, could improve soil functions such the aggregation of soil particles to give the soil better structure. This very large pool of carbon has seldom been considered even today as investigators produce carbon budgets in a climate change scenario, yet it seems key to me in getting a proper understanding of carbon flow in ecosystems irrespective of the plants or trees present in those environments. When I moved to Horticulture Research International (HRI) at Littlehampton in 1983, John Whipps joined me a year later and we extended our ideas of how microbes and plant interact around plant roots. I edited a book on *The Rhizosphere* in 1990. We particularly addressed at Littlehampton how microbes in the rhizosphere could control diseases. John with colleagues from Sheffield University coined the term of microbiome in 1988 when reviewing mycoparasitism around plants as a characteristic microbial community occupying a reasonably well-defined habitat which has distinct physicochemical properties. It was in 2001 that the Nobel laureate Joshua Lederberg extended these ideas to the human body in defining the microbiome as 'the ecological community of commensal, symbiotic and pathogenic microorganisms that literally share our body and space and have all but been ignored as determinants of health and disease'. The concept includes all microorganisms, including archaea, bacteria, eukaryotes, and viruses. Subsequently, the ideas have been applied to animals, plants, food environments, and biotechnology. Of particular interest has been the human gut (Figure 5.1). There has been a long history of the use of probiotics in the gut, especially *Lactobacillus acidophilus* as is used in yoghurt, to attempt to line the gut with a barrier against invasive pathogens. The success has been variable, but I have often seen benefits. In 2011 and 2013, the journal *Science* named the concept of the microbiome as the discovery of the year. In an article in Nature published on 3 February 2021, it was suggested that trillions of bacteria in the gut could have profound effects on the brain and used to halt a whole range of disorders, including Parkinson's disease, motor neurone disease, and Alzheimer's disease. Particularly,

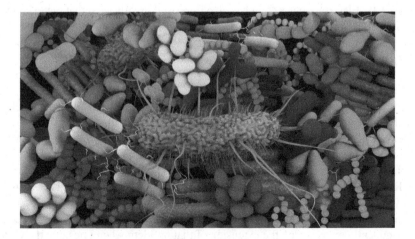

FIGURE 5.1 Microbiome of the human gut. (Getty Images.)

it was suggested that *Lactobacillus reuteri* could be used to disrupt the gut microbiome and treat autism spectrum disorder. Even though these early studies are largely with mice as models, it must offer much promise for the future to improve human life. In 2016, many of the US scientific and engineering societies came together to create the US Interdisciplinary National Microbiome Initiative in Washington DC, an event I was pleased to attend with Rita Colwell who had been one of the instigators. Investigation of microbiomes has been made easier by the capacity of modern genetic methods for detecting and characterising bacteria which includes DNA hybridisation, polymerase chain reaction (PCR), genetic sub-types, molecular epidemiology, ribotyping, and pulse-field gel electrophoresis. These may sound complicated but in practice, they are all methods for examining large pools of DNA quickly and relatively lower cost than in the past. As such it is much easier to investigate metagenomes which is the genetic material recovered from environmental samples. Since leaving her post as Director of the National Science Foundation, Rita has been chair of a company involved in metagenomic sequencing of microbiomes of the human gut. Pellets of faeces derived from healthy guts have been used to improve gut health of patients with gastrointestinal problems with very high success rates by a team at Massachusetts Institute of Technology. In the past, it was only possible for microbiologists to investigate what we now understand as microbiomes by isolating the microorganism with culture on an agar medium. The problem is that a very high proportion, perhaps 90%, of the organisms could not be cultured. One of the major advantages of DNA sequencing is that it does not require culture of the organisms. At the University of Surrey, we used high-throughput sequencing to investigate the composition and biodiversity of biofilms in wastewater treatment and found 108 genera of bacteria from the phyla Protobacteria, Bacteroides, and Firmicutes. The relative species composition was dependent on the temperature of operation. The study of the gut and the wastewater biofilm have some common ground as many of the species in the two environments are the same and ultimately, we must strive to build up populations that favour beneficial over harmful organisms. Wastewater analysis has been successfully used to monitor public health of communities, including the detection of COVID-19. Electron microscopy has also improved greatly such that pictorial representations of microbiomes can be seen more clearly and Figure 5.1 and the cover shows a microbiome from the gut. Microbiome analysis is relevant to all environments and reverting to the original description of the microbiome, it is highly relevant to plants where the aim is to develop the healthy microbiome around roots and shoots.

By analysing populations at the molecular level, the potential for gene exchange should be evaluated. When this was first considered in the UK, it was part of a wider consideration of introductions of new species of plants, animals, or microbes into a country. I joined the Interim Advisory Committee on Introductions (IACI) when it was set up in 1988, which subsequently became the Advisory Committee for Releases into the Environment (ACRE). In the initial mandate issues such as analysis of the spread of rhododendrons as a non-native species into the UK so that it spread rapidly to reduce the potential of land for farming, especially in hill country. I subsequently experienced the extension of that problem when I became the CEO of the Forestry Commission Research Agency in 2003; in that rhododendron provided the major host and vector for the spread of the sudden oak death (SOD) caused by the fungus *Phytophthora ramorum* and which was devastating in its impact. The only sensible and effective route we could pursue was the removal of rhododendron in many areas at massive cost. Subsequently, ash decline caused by the fungus *Hymenoscyphus fraxineus* entered the UK. The initial research strategy was to breed disease-resistant trees but that is a lengthy process whether classical or molecular methods are used. I wrote a letter to *The Times* on 30 October 2012 to suggest that a better understanding and management of the disease could be approached by using very high-resolution satellite imagery to target the problem. In an article entitled 'Treedemic' in *The Economist* in October 2021, it was indicated that millions of British trees have died from diseases and millions more will. With the creation of ACRE after IACI, the focus became the analysis of risks imposed by the deliberate release of genetically engineered microorganisms and plants into the environment, as opposed to involuntary introductions.

With my colleague Mark Bailey from the Centre for Ecology and Hydrology, we became the first to appear before ACRE to release a free living genetically modified microorganism, *Pseudomonas fluorescens*, into the environment. The bacterium was only modified with marker genes as a test case to monitor its spread and any possible gene transfer and assess any impacts on the environment and wheat grown at the HRI at Littlehampton in West Sussex, and on sugar beet grown at Wytham Wood, the University Field Station in Oxford. In papers published in *Nature Biotechnology*, we showed that the bacterium could spread 2 m from an inoculated wheat seed, that it could stay in the soil and colonise a crop the following year. The ecological fitness of the strain in soil was reduced by the genetic load of the marker genes but restored when it colonised the crop planted the following year. Importantly, there was no gene transfer to indigenous organisms detected or any adverse effect on crop or soil, or on human health. In other studies, with Fergal O'Gara in Cork University supported by the European Commission, we studied the effectiveness of a non-GM modified *P. fluorescens* strain which produced the antibiotic 2,4-diacetylphloroglucinol as a biocontrol agent for sugar beet diseases, and again that had no adverse effect on soil enzyme activities. Gene transfer from such bacteria might be more of a problem if they contained extrachromosomal DNA elements known as plasmids. Such plasmids can code for resistance to heavy metals and antibiotics. In the state of Maharashtra in India, I found water treatment plants with high concentrations of antibiotics and heavy metals, the latter resulting from the lack of prescription need and overuse. It is likely that antibiotic resistance was coded on plasmids in the microbiome of the wastewater, possibly on the same plasmid as heavy metal resistance, which might explain why the Indian population has such a high incidence of antibiotic resistance.

Biocontrol bacteria have not been exploited greatly by the agrochemical industry. A notable exception, however, is the insect parasitic nematodes, which release *Xenorhabdus* bacteria when they absorb them through orifices. This process was developed at HRI Littlehampton and now produced in the town by the agrochemical company BASF in 20 fermentation vessels generating 40 trillion nematodes. Extensive studies at HRI over many years also showed the capacity of the bacterium *Bacillus thuringiensis* to control insect pests biologically by producing a crystal toxin.

The toxin production can be genetically modified, and the gene has been inserted into plants, such as cotton to control boll weevil larvae and which is exploited commercially, even though there have been some concerns in India particularly that some beneficial insects could be affected. One strain of the bacterium could even kill mosquitos, although it has generally been considered that malaria control by this means would be uneconomic. Baculoviruses have been deployed with due consideration to environmental factors which govern their survival, especially in forests. Diseases have also been controlled successfully. The classic early successes were the control of crown gall of fruit trees and roses using the bacterium *Agrobacterium tumefaciens*, and the control of root rot of pine by the fungus *Peniophora gigantea*. These control processes, along with many other potential applications for a range of crops and trees, are reviewed in the book I edited with John Hobbie in *Microorganisms in Action*. Such approaches seemed to be a great way of producing healthy crops without loading the environment with chemicals described in Chapter 3. However, my comments made in 1988 were made with some caution because it was clear that the agrochemical industry felt threatened by this alternative to chemicals. Despite the extensive efforts on the International Organisation of Biological Control, the position today is that biocontrol practices have not been universally accepted or optimally utilised. The limitations to uptake have included risk-averse and unwieldy regulatory processes, increasingly bureaucratic barriers to access biocontrol agents, insufficient communication of the economic, and environmental benefits with the public and stakeholders which include growers and politicians. The biocontrol disciplines have also been fragmented. This is disappointing but could be remedied, and this will be considered again in the final chapter.

It was mentioned above that a bacterium applied to seed could be detected 2 m from the point of application. Release into the atmosphere could potentially give greater spread, especially if there is a wind. The science of aerobiology facilitates analysis of spread. Much study has been of fungi, but bacteria are also studied. Many studies have been undertaken on the spread of plant pathogens, sometimes by collecting them on samplers. I have seen this approach used at BRE Group near Slough in the UK, where samplers were used in underground train carriages and aircraft cabins located on site for experimental purposes. The information gained was confidential to the transport companies commissioning the work but almost certainly led to the installation of HEPA filters for aircraft cabins, even though they are not fully effective in taking out microbes, especially viruses. In the laboratory systems, experiments are made easier with genetic markers for tracking. There has been much less study of viruses. The other option is to look at the disease progression geographically in relation to meteorology. For example, SOD mentioned above has a very high incidence in the Pacific Northwest of the United States. When I made a field trip to investigate this, it was clear to me that the foggy conditions on the Pacific coast, while I was there, generated ideal conditions for disease on the infected trees close to the sea to spread inland over distances of several miles, but this would, of course, be by spread from tree to tree. Under these conditions, it should be possible to generate conceptual, empirical, simulation, synoptic, or regression mathematical models to study the epidemiology of the disease. Good models are now available to forecast potato late blight caused by the fungus *Phytophthora infestans*. Such information would have been invaluable to reduce the impact of the disease and prevent the Irish Potato Famine which ran from 1845 to 1852. It was clearly an epidemic but because it had appeared in the United States before Ireland, it could be termed a pandemic. Interestingly, when I investigated the 1 million deaths caused by the famine, it seems that many victims died from TB, largely as a secondary factor in the starvation as the human immune system had been compromised. A similar situation occurs with human immunodeficiency virus (HIV) where many patients die from TB and pneumonia from being immunocompromised. As a positive consequence of such a tragedy, many of those who escaped the famine by emigrating generated a new world order of Irish influence, especially in the United States where so many eventually contributed so much to so many spheres of life.

Pandemics can be spread through water as well as on land. One of the lead investigators of cholera has been Rita Colwell which is described in her book with Sharon Bertsch McGrayne in 2020 *A Lab of One's Own. One Woman's Personal Journey through Sexism in Science*. About 1.3–4 million cases and 21,000–143,000 deaths are recorded annually according to the World Health Organisation. Provision of safe water and sanitation are critical, and the diarrhoeal disease can kill within hours if left untreated. It is caused by the bacterium *Vibrio cholerae*, and environmental factors control the virulence, transmission, and epidemiology of the gastrointestinal disease. There are seasonal variations in disease occurrence, and this is linked to the presence of the crustacean copepods and phytoplankton blooms. From all the evidence, remote sensing using satellite imagery of the chlorophyll pigments and computer processing can be used to predict cholera outbreaks. This allows public health measures to be taken prospectively rather than retrospectively to control this historic scourge of mankind and ultimately prevent global pandemics of the disease.

One of the worst epizootic pandemics to reach UK agriculture was the foot-and-mouth disease (FMD) caused by a picornavirus, causing sores and blisters on the foot, mouth, and tongue of infected sheep, cattle, and pigs in 2001, which was mentioned in Chapter 1. The disease spread through Europe, especially Ireland and the Netherlands. There had been a previous outbreak in the UK in 1967. The first diagnosis of the 2001 outbreak was on 19 February at an abattoir in Essex, but the main source was thought to be in Northumberland where the disease had been concealed. The disease was exacerbated by the transport of animals and carcasses round the country and claims were made that the UK Government acted far too slowly to contain the disease which lasted until 30 September. Professor Neil Ferguson of Imperial College produced mathematical and epidemiological models for the UK Government which predicted that 15,000 animals would die. In practice, less than 200 died because the disease was largely contained by slaughter of infected animals as it was deemed that a vaccine could not act fast enough to contain spread. On route to Cumbria, which was the hardest hit region, I was contacted by the BBC News at 6 pm for a live interview for the opening feature to seek my opinion of the handling of the slaughtered animals which were being buried in unlined and unvented pits. While supporting the burials to contain the spread of disease, I pointed out the fallacy of the lack of lining not preventing passage of the disease by leaching, and gaseous emissions, which would include methane, that would ensue being potentially explosive. This was an example of failure to take a fully holistic approach to disease management. The cost to the economy was estimated to be £86 million, which included a reduction in tourism. However, what left a lasting impression on me was the impact on the mental health of the farming community, who were often poorly compensated for loss, and often resulted in suicides.

Even though FMD was of relatively short duration, and it was animals rather than humans directly impacted, the handling of the pandemic had much in common with COVID-19. Particularly we were unprepared nationally and globally. Mark Honigsbaum in his 2019 book *The Pandemic Century. A History of Global Contagion from the Spanish Flu to Covid-19* describes the epidemics we have been subjected to. Probably, the worst was the Spanish influenza pandemic caused by the H1N1 influenza A virus in 1918 and lasted for 2 years. A total of 500 million people, about a third of the world's population, were infected and there were 50 million deaths. No vaccines were available and non-pharmaceutical intervention included isolation, quarantine, personal hygiene, disinfectants, and limits to public gatherings. In 2003, there was an outbreak of severe acute respiratory syndrome (SARS), although it probably originated in 2002, in China. It was a 'super-spreader' coronavirus and moved to four other countries. The incubation period was 2–7 days. A total of 8098 cases were reported with 774 deaths. There was no cure or vaccine but was under control by July 2003. It appears that those who are infected and survive develop antibodies to further infection.

Although there had been an epidemic of Ebola virus disease around the Ebola River in the Democratic Republic of Congo in 1976, a country which remains vulnerable to the disease, the disease reached epidemic levels in West Africa (Liberia, Sierra Leone, Guinea) in 2014 and lasted until 2016. It was a zoonotic with bats as the primary transmission suspect. Five strains have been identified, four which affect people and one nonhuman primates. It is spread by body contact only. There is no medication or vaccine and the deaths reported at 11,323 represented a 90% mortality. The epidemiologist Professor Chris Witty who was then Chief Scientific Advisor to the Department for International Development in the UK said that the response to the disease was far too slow. Rene Dubos, a highly respected microbiologist at the Rockefeller Institute in New York had warned of the coming disease Armageddon, which could be made worse by mutation, and so in some ways these diseases were not total surprises. In 1958, he observed 'microbial disease is one of the inevitable consequences of life in a world where nothing is stable'. In 1977, he made his famous statement 'Think Globally, Act Locally'. Most of the research by Dubos was on combatting bacterial disease, but his comments are just as relevant to fighting disease induced by viruses. Nevertheless, nothing prepared us for the outbreak of COVID-19 in 2020 which originated in Wuhan, China, although there had been some warnings of dangerous pathogens in bat caves in China as far back as 2013. Bats themselves have a good immune response to virus infections. We still do not know however with any confidence if bats or any other animals were the transmitters of the disease. An excellent introduction to the disease was written by Michael Moseley in 2020 *Covid-19. What You Need to Know about the Coronavirus and the Race for the Vaccine*. The virus is relatively simple and has a core of a single strand of ribonucleic acid (RNA). Its outer membrane has club-like spikes which get into our cells and lock onto the ACE2 enzymes which play an important role in controlling blood

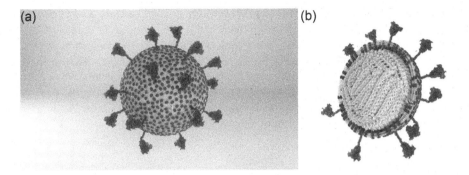

FIGURE 5.2 COVID-19. This shows the whole (a) and half (b) of the virus. The virus is about 0.1 μm in diameter, about one-tenth of the size of the average bacterium and about one hundredth the size of a plant or animal cell.

pressure (Figure 5.2). The body can find it difficult to detect and deploy its immune system. It is spread largely by coughs and sneezes and a major problem is that people who are infected often do not show symptoms even though they can spread the disease as asymptomatic carriers. This means that it can easily be spread by flights around the world. Viruses travel on fluid droplets and a single cough can release 3000 droplets travelling at 50 mph and release 200 million virus particles into the air, but some will fall to the ground. At 2 m, large droplets will be avoided, but if the particles are dispersed as aerosols they go much further as does cigarette smoke. A major difference to the SARS-CoV-2 virus is that whereas it can travel like COVID-19, it binds much better to ACE2 receptors and is therefore more infective. The clinical symptoms of COVID-19 are well described in Moseley's book, including aspects such as gender where men, older people, and black and ethnic minority groups are more likely to get sick and die.

The first alarm on COVID-19 was on December 31, 2019, when China informed the World Health Organisation (WHO) about 'a pneumonia of unknown cause' in Wuhan, a city of 11 million people. The next day 175,000 left the city after holidays to travel within China and abroad. After 10 days a death of a 61-year-old man from a novel coronavirus was reported and within 2 days the Chinese amazingly announced the full genetic blueprint of the virus which they shared with the rest of the world. Isolated cases were reported globally and on January 31 the WHO declared this outbreak a 'public health emergency of international concern'. It took until March 11 for the WHO to acknowledge that the spread of the virus was out of control and the world was in the grip of a serious pandemic. The severity of the disease varied between countries and actions taken also differed. For example, it took until March 23 for Boris Johnson to put the UK into lockdown. The lead committee for the UK was the Scientific Advisory Group for Emergencies (SAGE). Inputs to the committee had a strong dominance of mathematical modelling and epidemiology. For example, on March 26, a team led by Neil Ferguson (who had worked on FMD) suggested that social distancing measures could cut deaths globally from 40 million to less than 10 million. These measures were largely accepted globally in various ways but too early to analyse how valid the modelling was. Management by testing for infection, with consequent isolations, has been important using both the RAPID lateral flow immunological test and the test for COVID-19 DNA using the PCR. The PCR test is more expensive and more reliable than the RAPID test, but both can give false positive or false negative results. As a feat of scientific progress, the concept of the PCR test which was discovered by Kary Mullis in 1983, and for which he was awarded the Nobel Prize in Chemistry in 1993, would have been prohibitively expensive to use on such a large scale until recent times.

Moseley has been a champion of improving health by boosting the immune system by holistic means which include

- Shrink your waist
- Try intermittent fasting
- Eat a more Mediterranean-style diet
- Boost your microbiome
- Improve your sleep
- Become more active
- Reduce stress

From my own experience as Dean of a Biomedical School with a large Nutrition Department, these means all make sense and in my opinion a supplement like vitamin D can be important as so many people are deficient. Just how effective all this could be is still unclear but most of us, including Moseley, considered that a vaccine is the only effective measure. The only problem is that most people with any background in the area, particularly the UK Government's Chief Scientific Advisor Sir Patrick Vallance, a clinician who had previously been Chief Scientist to one of the world's leading pharma companies Glaxo Smith Kline, saw that even with a fair wind behind the science the regulatory barriers with trials would mean that a vaccine would take at least 18 months to develop. A further complication was that there are several variants of the virus because of its mutations. Under the new WHO scheme, it developed the variants of concern from 2020 and countries of the first detection are:

Alpha	UK	*Iota*	USA
Beta	South Africa	*Kappa*	India
Gamma	Brazil	*Lambda*	Peru
Delta	India	*Omicron*	South Africa
Eta	Nigeria, UK		

Of these, the *Delta* virus had been the most infective and caused the greatest concern, but *Omicron* is now more infective although less harmful.

Many countries joined the race to develop a vaccine which became possible when the DNA profile of SARS-Cov-2 was released by the Chinese authorities. The first to get approval was the Pfizer-BioNTech vaccine on December 11, 2020. It delivers a tiny piece of genetic code (mRNA) from the SARS-CoV-2 virus to boost host cells in the body to make these produce the spike protein, stimulating an immune response if the body is infected with the virus. The Moderna vaccine is an mRNA vaccine like the Pfizer-BioNTech product; both need to be stored in a freezer and therefore they are more difficult to transport. The Oxford-Astra Zeneca uses an engineered but harmless adenovirus (like the common cold) from chimpanzees to carry the spike protein to cells. It is like the Johnson & Johnson vaccine, and both can be stored in a refrigerator. The Novavax vaccine as a protein adjuvant contains the spike protein of the virus itself formulated as a nanoparticle which does not cause disease. Sputnik is also an adenovirus. Conventional vaccines take about 10–15 years to bring to market. The mRNA vaccines could be produced within a week, one of the massive advantages of modern molecular biology and chemistry. Synthetic production means no virus is needed. Vials of DNA with the spike protein contained on a plasmid are produced at −150°C. The plasmids are then put into the bacterium *Escherichia coli*. The bacterium is grown in a fermenter; the bacteria are then broken open with enzymes to release the plasmids, and the DNA purified by filtration. A single vial can give 50 million doses. For the adenovirus vaccines, infected cells are grown in bioreactors and purified after 60 days.

Even though the mRNA and adenovirus vaccines are produced much quicker than conventional vaccines, there is still a massive challenge to overcome, not only to get the vaccines produced and get through regulators, anti-vaccine resistance movements and combat the ever-increasing threat to human life globally. The book by Sarah Gilbert and Catherine Green *Vaxxers. The Inside Story of the Oxford AstraZeneca Vaccine and the Race against the Virus* published in 2021 is a fascinating detailed account of how this was achieved in less than 12 months. It is a detailed account of how the science and technology were developed but also a deeply personal account of the joys and frustration of their work. They also talk about the anti-vaxxers and ask the question as to why anyone would be ideologically opposed to a safe and cost-effective public health measure that saves millions of lives and stop people having to live with long-term disabilities that can be caused by diseases such as polio, small-pox, and COVID-19. What is more understandable is vaccine hesitancy and for that effective communication is vital to satisfy the concerns of the public about any risks, especially as many people are not familiar with risk analysis even in simplest terms like flying, driving, or walking along the street. They spell out clearly the effective collaboration they developed with their industrial partner, which has commonly been a cause of failure in the exploitation of discovery. It also details how effectively they worked with Andrew Pollard, the Chief Investigator of the Oxford-led clinical trials along with his team. In the past, Oxford had often failed to develop interdisciplinary collaboration but at this important time, they triumphed fast and flexibly with very effective management. That should not disguise the fact that the clinical trials could have been even more effective funding. It also needs to be recognised that so many of the team were on short-term funding (usually 3 years), and whereas they happened to be in place at the time of need, they will not necessarily be in place for Disease 'X' when it inevitably comes unless there is careful planning at the national and global level. It was also a triumph for women as in the past Rita Colwell in her book outlines the struggles women in science have often struggled to be accepted. That problem has been foreign to me as the teams I have managed have always had a gender balance on successes at all levels. For example, one of my successors as Dean of Biomedical Sciences at Surrey was Lisa Roberts. I recruited her before she completed her PhD studies in virology, she went on to become Dean and create a Veterinary School within the faculty with a focus on epizootic disease, which she assured me correctly that they would be the principal threats to human life in the future, and is now President of Exeter University.

The story of the development of the Pfizer-BioNTech vaccine is just as exciting as the Oxford AstraZeneca vaccine by Özlem Türeci with her husband Ugur Sahin. They cooperated with Joe Miller to write the book *The Vaccine: Inside the Race to Conquer the COVID-19 Pandemic.* Initially, Pfizer turned down the offer of developing the vaccine by the couple's company they founded in an unfashionable part of Germany because the company's top executives thought the virus would be rapidly contained like SARS and MERS, a view shared by many others at that time. Pfizer also thought that it might be too experimental. The couple persisted and produced the mRNA vaccine on a large scale effectively, bringing massive profits to both companies, while pricing it at 'cost of goods' for low-income countries. The couple sees that mRNA vaccines could be used for conditions such as cancer, but they would like to invest some of their profits into a malaria jab which is one of the most infectious diseases in the world, affecting so many small children. Even with the relative success of the vaccines against COVID-19, far too many people are hospitalised or die from the infection. It is important that there is an antiviral treatment against the disease. There are not many antivirals available but George Painter, who developed the mainstay drug treatment for HIV at the end of last century, has now developed Molnupiravir against COVID-19 and the UK is the first country to prescribe it.

It was mentioned in the Introduction that microbes could not only pose a threat in disease outbreaks, but that they might also be exploited offensively as weapons. Many countries have maintained research facilities to combat bioterrorism. In the UK, this was at Microbiological Defence Establishment at Porton Down in Wiltshire, originally attached to the Ministry of Defence. Many famous UK microbiologists worked there, including my own PhD supervisor John Pirt, and John Postgate who describes work there in his biography published in 2013 *Microbes, Music and Me. A Life in Science.* In 1942, 80 sheep were taken to the uninhabited Gruinard Island off the Scottish coast and bombs filled with anthrax (*Bacillus anthracis*) exploded over the 176 hectares. The bacterium forms spores which aid its survival and make it an ideal candidate for bioterrorism. It will infect grazing animals and usually causes death. It can infect humans as well. The experiment at Gruinard proved the capability of the bacterium as a weapon. In 1986, the land was decontaminated by spraying 280 tonnes of formaldehyde diluted in 2000 tonnes of seawater. I was contacted shortly after by William Stewart who was then Secretary of the Agricultural Research Council, but subsequently UK Government Chief Scientific Adviser, as to how I as a soil microbiologist would judge whether it was safe for people to return to the island. We agreed a plan and in 1990, it was declared safe and there have been no subsequent issues. In 2001, following the 9/11 attacks in Washington, the United States felt they would be threatened by further terrorist attacks. Rita Colwell attended a meeting of the CIA's Intelligence Science Board, both as the NSF Director and as an expert on bioterrorism. The information is still classified but it was learnt on October 7th that a man in Florida, Robert Stephens, had died from inhalation of anthrax, the first case in the US since 1975. Suddenly, on October 12th, a letter to NBC news anchor Tom Brokaw was opened by an office worker in New York and she saw a whitish-grey powder with the message 'This is next, take penicillin now, death to America, death to Israel, Allah is great'. So it started the sequence of what became 'The Anthrax Letters'. Rita was in an ideal position to take the lead in analysing and controlling the threat which she describes in her book. Many of us were contacted about the threat to provide any inputs we could make to the investigation. It became clear that it would be important to harness modern molecular techniques to identify dangerous pathogens, in the same way that it has been necessary those coming in a pandemic, if future threats are to be contained. It is also essential that any attempts to genetically modify organisms to generate harmful effects are controlled and contained. Such actions need to be driven by politicians on advice of scientists, but they must be ethical.

6 Bioethics and Governance

Ethics is knowing the difference between what you have a right to do and what is right to do.

Potter Stewart 1915–1985

A nation that destroys its soils destroys itself. Forests are the lungs of our land, purifying the air and giving fresh strength to our people.

Franklin D. Roosevelt 1882–1945

Governance is the strategic task of setting the goals of the organisation or government, with directions, limitations, and accountability frameworks. Management is the allocation of resources and oversight of the day-to-day operation of an organisation. Throughout my career in science, both as an experimentalist and as a manager and governor, most of my activity has been focussed on supporting policy nationally and internationally to improve life and the environment. As such most experiments in the laboratory and in the field have been subjected to ethical scrutiny which has given me reassurance to continue.

In the UK, there has been increased acknowledgement of the need for scientific advice in the development of government policy. The first UK Chief Scientific Advisor (CSA) was Solly Zuckerman who served from 1964 to 1971. Although the main function of the advisor has been to report to the Prime Minister, I have found them very approachable and enjoyed good relations with William Stewart (1990–1995), Robert May (1995–2000), and David King (2000–2008). The appointment of the current incumbent Patrick Vallance who was appointed in 2018 has been particularly timely during pandemic as he has a medical background and commercial experience in the pharma sector. All government departments now have a CSA, and they meet in a committee chaired by the government CSA. Generally, the CSAs are supported by expert committees. It does mean that to realise the potential of the UK that the government needs to increase spending in line with supportive words. In a comment in *The Times* in October 2021, Adam Smith, President of the Royal Society, pointed out that the UK produces 15.3% of the world's most highly cited papers but is only spending 1.7% of its gross domestic product of research which compares unfavourably with countries of the Organisation for Economic Development (OECD) overall (2.5%), United States (3.1%), and Germany (3.2%). Joe Biden has committed an additional $250 billion. The United States, the European Union, and most states now have analogous structures. The OECD has a range of committees to provide advice to its 38 member countries but has no regulatory function. In my experience that can potentially increase its influence.

Prime Ministers are commonly contacted by OECD headquarters in Paris to receive policy advice which is normally accepted. For example, two 'blue books' were produced by the organisation on how to safely release genetically modified organisms and most countries used this as the basis for national regulations. It is also useful to have more informal debate on how science may be used. In the UK, the Foundation for Science and Technology meets regularly to discuss topics of current interest and is attended by scientists from academia and industry, politicians, investors, diplomats, and public servants to listen to three presentations on an area of interest, followed by debate before and after a drinks reception and dinner. Debates are under Chatham House rules where nobody's comments are attributed so that debate can be freer and more open. I have enjoyed these sessions over many years with their facility to develop networks to aid the exploitation of science and technology. Until recently, the Chair of the Foundation was the Earl of Selborne, who had chaired many scientific committees and organisations, including the Parliamentary Scientific Committee. I had known John as a friend for most of my career and valued his support and guidance when he visited me in most organisations I had worked in; his passing in 2021 was a great personal loss to me.

Some people get sceptical about engaging with big business and hedge funds on ethical grounds, yet they can be key to the exploitation of science and technology, often by philanthropy. For example, the Bill and Melinda Gates Foundation has made major investments in healthcare, especially malaria control, and innovative agriculture in Africa. Paul Tudor Jones, American billionaire and one of the world's most successful hedge funders, is helping to transform Africa's conservation movement. He has a simple formula: find a place that's unloved, and provide capital, and try to convert it to ecotourism. Jones has also become a legendary fundraiser in the US for the disadvantaged of New York through his Robin Hood Foundation, which recently helped to raise $110 million in an hour for those hit hardest by COVID. My own travels in Africa in recent years, in part as a board member of the Council for the Frontiers of Knowledge, have made me realise how much reward there can be in supporting counties in development, especially in the field of conservation. The UN Biodiversity Conference was held in China in October 2021, and even though it had less attention than COP 26 in Glasgow in November 2021 but its global impact is large and interlinked with climate change.

For many people, the definition of bioethics focuses on the study of ethical, social, and legal issues that arise in biomedicine. In my mind, this should be extended to cover an analysis of all processes in the biosphere which affect life, especially those taking place in the environment, such as climate change. This approach is taken by John Bryant and Linda La Velle in their book *Introduction to Bioethics* published in 2019. Bioethics relates to most natural, physical, and social sciences. Religious and theological thinking can be brought to bear on bioethics and is an aspect of moral theology. The quotations above by the former President of the United States and the former Associate Justice of the Supreme Court of the United States are apposite to our thinking on how life should be governed. Bioethics should support governance and policy making but unfortunately is often ignored. This can lead to trust being challenged, a topic which is covered by Glynis Breakwell in her book published in 2021 *Mistrust*. Trust is a social psychological process. Although there are many definitions of trust, it commonly refers to holding a firm belief in reliability, honesty, strength, or ability of someone or something. Mistrust focuses on being suspicious of someone or something, upon being doubtful, wary, or full of misgivings. Distrust is more unidimensional: the feeling that someone or something cannot be relied upon to be truthful or to behave as they are supposed to. Hazards generate risks and mistrust is intimately interlinked to these. Rumours can be spread by social media, leading to a disinformation crisis, a technique practised by Donald Trump during his presidency, especially related to COVID-19. This can result in conspiracy theories. SARS-CoV-2 was a dream for conspiracy theorists because of uncertainty, fear, and personal threat. The task of Anthony Fauci, Chief Medical Advisor to the President of the United States and a specialist in infectious disease, to tackle this has been massive and he includes this in a 2022 book on his life *Fauci-Expect the Unexpected: Ten Lessons on Truth, Service, and the Way Forward*, which is drawn from interviews for the film *Fauci* by *National Geographic Documentary Films* which streams on Disney+. The problem with COVID-19 is that:

- It arrived out of the blue – no slow-burn anticipation of disaster.
- It spread rapidly.
- It could spread by people who were not symptomatic.
- It killed indiscriminately and painfully.
- It was not controlled by existing vaccines.
- It drove whole nations into a state of self-imposed paralysis.
- It evoked the basis for a panoply of dystopic fears surrounding the curtailment of civil liberties in attempts to curtail the virus.
- It laid waste to the global economy.
- It mutated many times to become more virulent just as vaccines were rolled out to contain it.

For conspiracy theories to be effectively managed, policy makers should benefit from the input of social scientists.

One of the first bioethical considerations for many people will have been a discussion in a hospital when an ageing relative is nearing the end of life. One option may be for the patient to enter a hospice for care and continue life in a dignified manner adding 'life to the time left'. Care is patient-centric, neither trying to extend nor shorten life. It accepts dying and accompanies the patient on that journey, minimising the unpleasant and optimising the pleasant aspects. Medical staff may decide to authorise a 'Do Not Resuscitate' order on the patient in a hospital or hospice while ensuring that the patient remains pain-free. Whereas relatives are usually consulted so that the views of the patient can be considered, no one patient or relative has the right to demand any specific treatment, although they can refuse any treatment or intervention. This contrasts with a euthanasia request from somebody who is not at the end of life but who prefer to end their lives because of their medical state. Fortunately, in most countries, assisted dying is still illegal but there will be an ongoing bioethical and legal debate. The view of the Church is clear in that innocent life should be protected and I support that view while having full sympathy for those who are severely disabled.

Bioethical debate is just as relevant to the start of life, especially through the route of *in vitro* fertilisation. The English moral philosopher Mary Warnock chaired the inquiry in the UK to create the Human Fertilisation and Embryo Act of 1990 where a legal framework was set that governs infertility treatment and medical services ancillary to infertility treatment such as embryo storage which now legally allows infertile women to give birth. Most religions and Christian faiths approve of this, but the Catholic Church has expressed reservations. The 1987 Doctrine of Faith *Donum Vitae* (Instruction on respect for human life in its origin and on the dignity of procreation) teaches that if a given medical intervention *helps* or *assists* the marriage act to achieve pregnancy, it may be considered moral; if the intervention *replaces* the marriage act to engender life, it is not moral. Of greatest concern has been the disposal of any fertilised embryos which subsequently have to be discarded. One argument is that these could be used for women who cannot afford normal IVF treatment, which is expensive, although seems somewhat impracticable. It seems inevitable that the debate will continue. One aspect of this is the issue of vaccines which come from human foetal cells at some stage to produce vaccines for rubella, hepatitis A, and chickenpox. Even the successful Oxford-AstraZeneca vaccine for COVID-19 had one line from chicken but another from a foetal kidney cell aborted in 1973. The judgement of the Catholic Church in the pandemic is that people should follow their own conscience on whether to receive that vaccine, although, in practice, in the UK people were not given a choice of vaccines they would receive and immunity against the virus sensibly seemed to of paramount importance. As we get more disease threats, more vaccines will be necessary and this will keep the bioethical debate in focus amongst those with genuine concerns, but also sadly with the anti-vaxxers. It is important that ethically derived cell lines should be made available for vaccine development.

In the 1990s, I taught an interactive course to a large biosciences class on the ethics and implications of genetic engineering. While recognising the potential of gene editing, most students' biggest fear was that it would get out of control leading to designer babies. Emmanuelle Charpentier, a French microbiologist was investigating the ancient immune system CRISPR/Cas of the bacterium *Streptococcus pyogenes* which causes numerous infections in humans and discovered a molecule called tracrRNA that cleaves viral DNA. In 2011, she met with Jennifer Doudna from California, and they realised they could harness this action in gene editing as a form of genetic scissors for rewriting the code of life and potentially change the world. This led to the award of the Nobel Prize in Chemistry in 2020 to Charpentier and Doudna. Ironically, He Jiankui in China used CRISPR genome editing to alter embryos which were implanted, and two children were born. This was not just bad science but textbook violation of ethics, for which he was jailed, and his laboratory closed. However, that having been carried out, an article in *Nature Biotechnology* in November 2021 argues that we could still learn something useful by tracking the health of the children that were born. Doudna feels that the first real applications of the CRISPR gene technology will be in agriculture, but it could have general applications in clinical medicine such as sickle cell disease, cancer-causing viruses, and even ageing. The technology can simply find a piece of DNA in a cell where there is now such a vast array of gene libraries and alter it by editing. This massive advance has so much potential to improve life directly and through the food we eat, but there are potentially more sinister implications in the production, for example, of the designer babies mentioned above. Clearly, bioethics has a major role to play in the way forward and we must hope that the global community will want to see tight regulation and control, as indeed do the investigators. As I write this (2 September 2021), there was a headline in *The Times* of London 'Britain to grow cancer-cutting wheat for making healthier bread'. The wheat has been genetically edited using CRISPR and will be grown at Rothamsted in the UK under approval from the UK government with its new flexibility under post-Brexit. The gene-edit reduces the level of the amino acid asparagine because it can be converted to acrylamide, which is thought to be carcinogenic. It was successfully argued that CRISPR modification is fundamentally different from conventional genetically modified crops because nothing is added, and the changes could have occurred by natural mutation. If the trials succeed, this will be one of the first examples of genetic modification of crops improving human health.

Whereas medicine has been the focus of much of the bioethics debate, people will not stay healthy if they do not have enough food. Food security therefore must be a major topic for bioethics and much of the world experiences food poverty, especially as the growth of the human population now exceeds the growth of agricultural production. In September 2021, the United Nations Secretary-General convened a Food Systems Summit, only the sixth such meeting since 1943, arguing that the food system needs a revamp because one in ten people in the world is undernourished, one in four is overweight, and more than one-third of the world's population cannot afford a healthy diet. Food supplies are disrupted by heatwaves, floods, droughts, and wars. Seven science-driven priorities were identified:

1. End hunger and improve diets
2. De-risk food systems
3. Protect equality and rights
4. Boost bioscience
5. Protect resources
6. Sustain aquatic foods
7. Harness digital technology

Trade tariffs and market protection by rich countries, the forcing of monoculture farming on poor economies, and gross wastage of food in the West are major causes of poverty and hunger in the developing world.

Clearly, one of the options as indicated by Doudna with the new technology is to genetically engineer crops to improve productivity, but at this stage, conventional genetic modification has been the route. The pioneer scientist in this arena in 1983 was Marc van Montagu who I had the pleasure to meet on several occasions at his laboratory at Gent in Belgium. He showed a bacterium *Agrobacterium tumefaciens* induced tumours in plants with a plasmid known as the Ti-plasmid and that this plasmid could be used as a vector to genetically modify plants. Van Montagu's group also investigated the modification of bacteria that lived around plant roots (the rhizosphere) which was the primary reason that I collaborated with him. It was not until

2013 that he became a recipient of the World Food Prize for this work. In between, there was extensive public debate and protest based on intrinsic objections, risk, lack of consumer choice, and wider social issues. It is right that risk be evaluated, but it was shown that there is no need for special containment in terms of gene flow and it is very unlikely that any antibiotic resistance could flow from the marker genes used in the constructs. It is also extremely unlikely that superweeds could be created by gene flow. Indeed, it seemed to me that genetic loading of the constructs likely reduces ecological fitness. One of the commercial companies to exploit the crops was Monsanto. I had extensive discussions with them, and I think they made a very bad mistake by inserting what they called a terminator gene into the GM crops to prevent seeds being saved by famers from season to season and they would have to buy new seed each year from the company. Particularly in developing countries, it is normal practice for farmers to save seeds and it seemed unethical to me to prevent this. The resulting public outcry nearly destroyed the commercial interest of the company and they had to support the farmers. Fortunately, there is now an international moratorium on the use of terminator genes. I introduced Monsanto to my psychologist colleague Glynis Breakwell who pointed out to them that the only way to move forward would be to use focus groups of consumers to get opinions and modify strategies, but we were unable at the time to convince them of the social science approach. The first commercial use of a GM crop was in 1996, and by 2016, there were 26 countries in which they were grown, amounting to about 12.3% of the world's arable land (about 185 billion hectares). The major countries are the United States, Brazil, Argentina, Canada, and India, but the uptake in the UK has been poor. In 2000, OECD organised the Conference on the Scientific and Health Aspects of Genetically Modified Foods. Because of my role in OECD, at the time I was summoned to Paris by Gerard Viatte (Director of Agriculture) for him to express his concerns to me that the British Prime Minister (Tony Blair) would try to force the issue for adoption of the crops instead of allowing full debate in line with OECD principles. I spoke to John Krebs who chaired the meeting to contain this, and he produced an excellent dispassionate report. Nevertheless, the adoption of the technology is down to consumer choice in a democratic society and the British public have continued to be reluctant. With all the interest in genetically modified crops, in recent times it is perhaps unfortunate that the interest in conventional plant breeding by selection has been diluted. This has served us well in the past and resulted in the green revolution, particularly in India. I had the great pleasure to meet in Mexico the Nobel Peace and World Food prizes winner Norman Borlaug who selected disease-resistant wheat. I also worked at Washington State University with Orville Vogel who selected short-stem wheat varieties that produced yield increases of 25%. It seems to me that plants selected in this way will often be ecologically fitter than those that are genetically modified and carry a genetic load.

Genetic modification is far from the only route to generate food security. One of the most important areas to consider is land use and land use change to get improved production from simple measures such as crop rotation as opposed to monocropping. However, some of these approaches can backfire especially when the motive is solely economic gain and no consideration of environmental and social consequences. The clearance of rainforests, particularly in Amazonia, has had land use change as the primary motive and especially land clearance for agriculture to produce soya to feed beef cattle. Clearly, this has a big impact on climate change, but it also has a massive direct impact on people. It was a great experience to visit Brazil to discuss this with native people and policy makers, but I have never engaged directly with the politicians who control the situation. We saw in Chapter 4 that meat production is in the long-term dubious in terms of global sustainability. Importantly, however, forest clearance destroys the livelihoods of indigenous people who are dependent on the forest for their livelihoods. Globally 1.2 billion people depend on forests for their livelihoods or one-fifth of the world's population. A problem is that much of the logging is illegal, amounting to 50%–90% of tropical production, and worth about US$30–100 billion annually. This has a big impact on trade, not just indigenous people, and consequently, the European Union, in association with the European Forest Institute launched a scheme Forest, Law, Enforcement, Governance and Trade, stated in 2003. It involves signing a Voluntary Partnership Agreement between the EU and the country at presidential level to prevent illegal logging and now amounts to a total of 15 countries. Clearly, trade is the driver but the knock-on effect to indigenous people is a bioethical advantage, although it is unfortunate that Brazil is not a VPA country. Indeed, President Bolsonaro has been very negative, preferring to concentrate on short-term commercial gains to his country, in part supported by the United States in the Trump era.

One of the other consequential bioethical concerns on cropping has been the use of crops to produce biofuel, diverting the land use from food and animal feed production. The ethical advantage is to reduce our dependence on fossil fuels. Perhaps somewhat ironically, the lead country has been Brazil when they created their National Alcohol Programme in 1975. This was a consequence of their poor balance-of-payments because of oil imports, heavily constraining the economy. The process was quite simple fermentation technology generating the alcohol from the sugars in sugar cane, just like the process to produce beer and wine. The fuel produced for cars is known as gasohol. The lipid components of some crops such as oilseed rape are used to produce biodiesel. This route is known as first-generation biofuels. If land use and food security concerns were not an issue, the prospect would be great for many countries, and I had the opportunity to visit Mexico and South Africa to discuss the issues with them. Issues occurred in the United States when former President Bush encouraged Mid-West farmers to use corn for biofuels increased prices. Cattle farmers could then no longer afford to buy the corn as feed and, therefore, might be considered an unethical political decision. I was asked by OECD to convene a workshop in 2007 on Bioenergy Policy Analysis at Umea in Sweden and concluded that the technique of Life Cycle Assessment was necessary in all cases to ensure that a holistic analysis of risks and benefits is made, sustainability is assessed, and the environment is not compromised. The debate was taken further at a meeting in Copenhagen the following year. In the UK, the Nuffield Council on Bioethics produced a report in 2011 *Biofuels. Ethical Issues* and recognised the moral imperative to reduce the consumption of fossil fuels, any development of biofuels should meet clear ethical standards. Second-generation biofuels avoided this issue by using waste plant materials such as the plant biomass left after the extraction of sugar from sugar cane and using enzyme fermentations which could use the cellulosic material. Similarly,

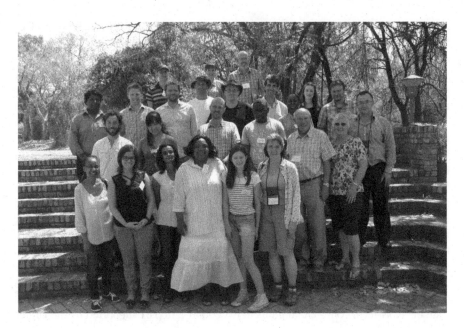

FIGURE 6.1 SUPERGEN Bioenergy Hub and University of Stellenbosch Workshop to discuss the potential of biofuels involving young British and South African scientists with senior mentors at Kruger National Park in 2014. Author is second from right on the second step.

third-generation biofuels avoid the use of agricultural land completely by using algae, and fourth-generation biofuels use bacteria and fungi such as yeasts. Brazil has continued to lead on biofuel production from sugar cane globally but there has been a decline in the number of cars produced using gasohol. It is important that there is international cooperation with teams at all levels as we appraise the opportunities of biofuels and indeed all aspects of science which can enhance sustainability of the planet, especially in rural communities (Figure 6.1). For example, on an EU-Funded trip to Ghana, we identified the opportunity for rural communities to produce power from the oil of the jatropha plant, which produces fewer environmental concerns than oil palm cultivation which reduces carbon capture by felling tropical forests, particularly in Southeast Asia. Such small-scale production of a biofuel could make power available to the community where it did not exist, enabling children to study in the evenings at home (Figure 6.2).

The Nuffield Council on Bioethics has reflected on COVID-19 and argues that bioethics should have played a critical role in pandemic response since the beginning. They ask how we balance different interests (individual and collective; economic and social) and different risks (the risks of morbidity and mortality of COVID-19; the risks of poor health associated with poverty and isolation)? Whose interests (the young, the elderly, the key workers) should have been given priority? On what basis and by whom, are these decisions being made? Transparency is essential. We hear that ethnic minority groups are more affected but how is that segregated from populations experiencing social deprivation? The Council argued that any public health measures should be evidence based and proportionate, and that should be communicated clearly to the public. They argue for two values: trustworthiness to gain the

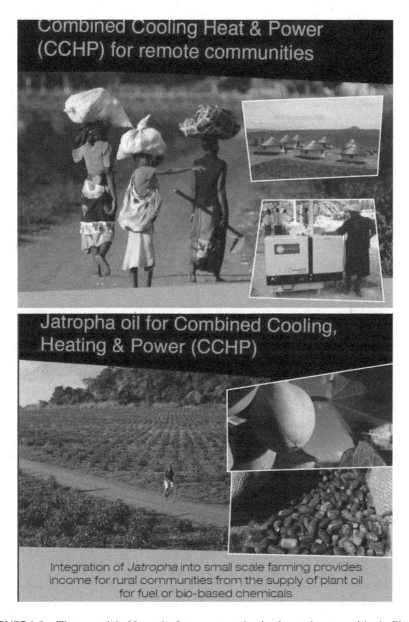

FIGURE 6.2 The potential of Jatropha for energy production in rural communities in Ghana.

support of the public and solidarity to generate sharing of burdens between individuals, between the state and individuals, and between countries. They argued that 'following the science' as the government kept announcing to justify policy decisions is not politically or morally neutral and it does not deliver policy answers that involve values and judgements for which people are responsible and should be scrutinised and accountable. Which values are in play and what judgements are being made? By whom? On what advice? Testing, certification, treatments, and vaccination are key policy issues. The nature and effectiveness of testing has been highly variable, as well as having sometimes unreasonable costs to travellers. However, immunity certification and passporting is likely to fall disproportionately on the disadvantaged. Vaccination has been effective in high-income countries generally but is barely started elsewhere which raises issues of global equity. One of the other big issues the Council has raised in its blogs is 'what is an acceptable level of death?', an issue which has also been covered by *Nature*. The government will not pick a number, even with winter flu as a comparator. We might accept an annual addition of 20,000 deaths from an endemic COVID-19, which in a bad year could rise 30,000, and some have even suggested figures as high as 50,000. This is shaped by statistical modellers who seem to be at the heart of the government decision-making in generating outcomes of policy options. Those inputs are important but even the government Deputy CSA, Angela McLean, has said that 'we really need a sensible discussion of what might be acceptable which is not just a scientific question but a question for the whole of society'. For public acceptability, we need total transparency. Ethics has regrettably not featured highly in government policy making during the pandemic, and it should be centre stage. Fundamental moral questions of the balance of loss of life against predicted gains should be analysed. It is not comparable with winter flu, especially considering the effects of 'Long COVID' and the indirect effects of living with such a serious pandemic. The acceptability of death cannot be determined by a balance of losses and gains that yields an optimal figure of overall casualties. There is also the issue of fairness and, for example, the Health Foundation found that 'those younger than 65 in the poorest 10% of areas in England were almost four times more likely to die from COVID-19 than those in the wealthiest'.

At the early stage of the COVID-19 pandemic, Ben Bramble, a philosophy lecturer at the Australian National University, produced a book in August 2020 *Pandemic Ethics. 8 Big Questions of COVID-19* which he made available freely on open access. Even though it was at an early stage, it gave a very good template for bioethical considerations. His eight questions are:

1. **Lockdown**: Should we stay locked down and wait for a vaccine, cure, or treatment, or open up in the hopes of achieving herd immunity without a vaccine?
2. **Blame**: Who is morally to blame for COVID-19 (both its genesis and spread)?
3. **Immunity passports**: Should we allow people who are immune to the virus to leave lockdown?
4. **Masks**: How should we respond to shortages of facemasks and other PPE?
5. **Duties to assist**: What positive moral duties do various parties have in a pandemic?
6. **Vaccine trials**: Should we allow people to volunteer to be exposed to SARS-CoV-2 to speed up the development of a safe and effective vaccine?
7. **Triage**: When hospitals run out of life-saving resources (e.g., ventilators, ICU beds, and dialysis machines); who should get their use?
8. **Onlookers**: How should those who are medically nor economically harmed by the pandemic live and feel in these times?

The moral issues are set out with possible answers. He points out that one of the most frightening aspects of COVID-19 is its ability to potentially lead to hospitals becoming overburdened or running out of vital resources. Physical distancing and good hygiene are obviously main routes to slow transmission. Citizens, including prisoners and protestors, rights are a clear issue. Algorithms that predict the expected number of years a patient has remaining are inevitably imperfect but can be improved. Partygoers can be the problem onlookers. A major moral argument is that if we accept non-essential workers should have the right to work during pandemic, the working lives of many of the underprivileged subsets must be improved after pandemic; politicians and policy makers need to act on this. To protect the world from future pandemics, we need better global surveillance, early suppression by social distancing, and increased support for vaccine development.

In the UK, the Scientific Committee Advisory Group for Emergencies (SAGE) took a key role in the COVID-19 pandemic, with Patrick Vallance (CSA) and Chris Whitty (Chief Medical Officer) as key players. An important member, until he resigned in November 2021, has been Jeremy Farrer who is Director of the Wellcome Trust, one of the world's leading funders of health research. He felt sufficiently concerned about the way government handled advice that he wrote a book with Anjana Ahuja in 2022 *Spike – The Virus v The People. The Inside Story.* Farrar is an expert on emerging infectious diseases and well respected so it is very concerning that he should speak so strongly against political leaders by suggesting that they rejected any science that did not suit their extreme libertarian ideology. He worries that he might be seen as complicit in the government's deadly mistakes with the government repeatedly ignoring the timely prescriptions for action by SAGE, with deaths resulting. A week's delay in the initial lockdown might cost about 20,000 lives. Their refusal is to lock down again in the autumn of 2020 when it was clear that it was needed probably caused tens of thousands more deaths and was unforgiveable. He calls Dido Harding's test and trace 'a grave error', and I agree with that view. It seems to me to have been highly flawed in concept and delivery. Farrar also feels that there should have been far less secrecy around SAGE, in part caused by pre-publication secrecy of vital information, and that there should have been better diagnosis, surveillance, vaccines, wildlife management with high-level global disease authority. He also suggests there were tensions between Patrick Vallance and Chris Witty who was wary of over-reacting to the threat. That is of course possible, but my own view is that Chris Witty who I have met had very relevant experience as a leading epidemiologist dealing with the Ebola outbreak in Africa, as well as being very effective in communication. Also, Patrick Vallance had an excellent background both as a leading clinician and academic, as well as having worked as a research director in the pharma sector. However, COVID-19 was a very different virus and its transmission and capacity to mutate can as a surprise to many people with expertise. As we have seen earlier in the book, it is normal in science for there to be debate between competent individuals and this is healthy.

Part of the problem for everybody was trying to get to the root of the COVID-19 outbreak in China. At the time, the threat of a bioterrorist act could not be ruled out, nor could unintentionally release from the Wuhan Institute of Virology. It seemed to me at the time that the disease had to be zoonotic, but it was a real challenge to get information, even by the World Health Organisation (WHO) team that was sent in. Some criticised the selection of the team because Peter Daszak, an expert on the ecological origin of viruses had links to the Institute. Also, the WHO had discussions in Beijing that gave the Chinese a veto on the selection of scientists in the mission. It was perhaps unfortunate for the WHO in terms of independence that the Director-General Tedros Adhanom Ghebreyesus was a long-term friend of China who had backed his candidacy strongly. China had a bad legacy with the 2003 SARS crisis, the first pandemic of the twenty-first century, when they deliberately prevented the release of information on infections and spread. It was agreed that the theory of virus escape would not be investigated. Everybody in China would have been worried about humiliation by admitting any guilt because of bad practice. But such things happen such as in Birmingham in 1978 when the smallpox virus escaped from a university laboratory, but the important thing is to learn from mistakes to avoid future occurrence. However, *The Times* reported in September 2021 that over 100 safety breaches have been investigated in UK laboratories that handle dangerous viruses and other pathogens in the past 15 years, and the real number is likely to be higher, making a leak by whatever means from the Wuhan laboratory seem quite possible. It is also possible that it could have been carried by a person from the laboratory and, of course, the initial source could still pass through the wet animal markets. The fact is that nobody is sure on what happened, but Peter Embarek, the Danish Scientist who led the WHO team that visited Wuhan in January 2021, said in August 2020 that a lab leak was a 'likely hypothesis', even though his team had rejected such a theory. Successive former US Presidents have expressed concerns on the handling of affairs in China and in March 2021, President Joe Biden asked his intelligence services to uncover the truth.

The US has been fortunate to have Anthony Fauci as Chief Medical Advisor to the President and a lead member of the White House Coronavirus Task Force. He is an outstanding physician-scientist, specialising in immunology and Director of the National Institute of Allergy and Infectious Diseases, who has had a robust but effective relationship with two presidents but importantly is an excellent communicator to the public. Certainly, it is important to restore public trust in the events which led to pandemic and in the management of the disease in all countries. In the UK, Susan Michie has pointed to the need for behavioural change in the pandemic and it is good for democracy that an independent SAGE to give weekly briefings was created with former CSA David King as a lead spokesperson. Governance vehicles during pandemic have varied greatly globally. For example, the cautious policies of Jacinda Ardern in New Zealand are in marked contrast with the cavalier approaches of the Brazilian President Jair Bolsonaro in Brazil. This is where international governance though bodies such as WHO are so important to attempt to get balance.

Whereas we look to governments and their associated bodies for leadership, many people look to their religious leaders for moral guidance. The environmental guidance by Pope Francis through *Laudato Si'* was mentioned in Chapter 4. It is clear that he had intended to play a significant role in COP 26, but it has been encouraging to read in September 2021 that he as leader of the Roman Catholic Church, along with the leader of the Eastern Orthodox Church (Patriarch Bartholomew), and the leader of the Anglican Communion (Archbishop Justin Welby) have come together for the first time to warn of the 'catastrophic consequences' of climate change in advance of COP 26. It would be good if the leaders of all religious faiths signed up to this initiative. There has been much development on the thinking on life in churches. For example, the Second Vatican Council (Vatican II) was one of the most significant events in attempting to modernise the life of the Roman Catholic Church, held in Rome between October 1962 and December 1965 under the call of Pope John XXIII to let some 'fresh air' into the Church. Churches and other religions should be thought just as important stakeholders as policy makers in the protection life. The volume which resulted *Gaudium et Spes. On the Church in the Modern World* introduced by Cardinal Angelo Scola in 1966 considered such topics as The Dignity of the Human Person, The Community of Man, The Concerns of Man in the World at Large, Social-Economic Life, and the Life of the Political Community. For many, the implementation of the ideas expressed is far too slow, and there is a new initiative to accelerate this in 2023 by the bishops, but, of course, there are also many who do not want to see change, amongst both clergy and lay people. There are also frustrations from many people about behaviour, such as abuse by clergy in all churches. Answers to these issues gain importance as society becomes increasingly secular. James Gerard McEvoy tackles these issues from a historical perspective in his 2014 book *Leaving Christendom for Good. Church-World Dialogue in a Secular Age*. It includes an analysis on the corruptions of modernity as the personal views of the Emeritus Pope Joseph Ratzinger. Most recently (September 2021), an article in *The Times* was captioned 'My Catholic critics hope that I will die, says the Pope', in which Pope Francis criticised those who sought security in the past, describing their 'rigidity' and 'clericalism' as the 'evil of the moment, and 'two perversions'. Of course, doctrine must be declared by all churches, and it should help people to believe in God. Unfortunately, it can often have the opposite effect. It has already been mentioned in Chapter 2 how people like Stephen Hawking and Roger Penrose have moved towards agnosticism or even atheism in frustration. In Paul Nurse's Book *What Is Life* (2021), he describes similar frustration by suggesting as a boy to his Baptist minister that when God was speaking about the Genesis account of creation, he was explaining what happened in terms that would make sense to an uneducated, pastoral population 2000 or 3000 years ago. Should it be treated more like a myth, but that, God had devised an even more wonderful mechanism for creation, by inventing evolution by natural selection. Unfortunately, the minister did not see that at all and told him that he had to believe the literal truth of Genesis and said that he would pray for him! That started his gradual descent from religious belief to atheism, or to be more precise, sceptical agnosticism. Of course, Nurse's views are consistent with those of Charles Darwin who suggested natural selection could take place without invoking a supernatural Creator, bringing him into conflict with the Church. However, Darwin believed in God as a First Cause and the ultimate lawgiver and as such considered himself a theist. These distinctive views can be rationalised as Darwin sustaining faith, by contrast to Nurse who in my opinion was alienated not even by dogma but the irrational analysis of a particular minister. Richard Dawkins, the distinguished Oxford evolutionary biologist, embraced Christianity in a normal Anglican upbringing until he reached 15 years of age. He then concluded that the theory of evolution alone was a better explanation for the complexity of life and ceased believing in a God. He expressed his doubts in 2006 in a book *The God Delusion* and followed this in 2019 with a book *Outgrowing God. A Beginner's Guide.* He has become a proponent of atheism, asserting the supremacy of science over religion in explaining the world. His writing is eloquent, very funny and he is a great thinker, which explains his position as a best-selling author of non-fiction. In defending his atheistic views, he describes the beauty of biology and evolution and argues that none of this requires a God and indeed, nobody has ever proved the existence of Christ or any other God. However, rigorous scientific analysis of his arguments does not seem to me to be proof on non-existence, any more than we can prove existence of God. Again, the position of faith must come into play to argue for the existence of God, which is not dependent on the dogma of religion. One of the greatest free-thinking philosophers of our time was Bertrand Russell, who published a series of essays in 1957 under the title *Why I Am Not a Christian.* Many of his views accord with those of Dawkins. The book also describes The Bertrand Russell Case of 1940 in which a malignant campaign succeeded in getting Russell 'unfit' to teach philosophy in New York College. Agree or not with his views, free speech should always be allowed and indeed in 2021, the UK government has found it necessary to restate the case for free speech in UK universities. A major opponent of the views of Dawkins is David Bentley Hart in the 2013 book *The Experience of God. Being, Conscious, Bliss.* He dissects most of his arguments from a theological standpoint. For example, he contests Dawkins's view that any creator of the cosmos would have to be very complex indeed, and since complexity is produced by evolution, the existence of such a being is vanishingly unlikely. This is a parody. As the notion that mechanically complex reality can be created only by something even more mechanically complex does not even follow the logic of mechanical causation, since a structurally simpler object can be the efficient cause of an object structurally more complex than itself. But, since mechanisms cannot create anything in the proper sense, because creation is the donation of existence to what has no existence, mechanical complexity is therefore of no relevance here at all. Indeed, all advanced theistic traditions insist that God is metaphysically simple. Dawkins's vision of God would be impossible as he would be both the product of nature and the creator nature, which means he would have to create himself, a very difficult feat!

One of Dawkins's opponents in debates in Oxford has been John Lennox, Emeritus Professor of Mathematics who produced the book in 2020 *Where Is God in a Coronavirus World*, in which he examines COVID-19 in the light of various belief systems and shows how the Christian worldview not only helps to make sense of it, but it also offers us real hope to cling to. Many theists respond to disasters like pandemics, earthquakes, and tsunamis by reaffirming their faith in God but others from various religions respond by arguing that the crisis is a direct judgement of God. The latter is irrational and has no basis in the Bible or other religious works. Similarly, the atheist approach using such judgement is of no help. Although Dawkins writes eloquently in describing biology and beauty in nature without the need for a God, his deterministic version of atheism abolishes the categories of good and evil, replacing them with blind indifference in a fatalistic universe. As such COVID-19 cannot be bad or evil and the Dawkins view would be simply rearrangement of atoms! Ironically, he considers that atrocities such as 9/11 are evil. For morality, in my opinion, we need an objective standard of good. Morality comes out of free will in humans. Removing God from the equation does not remove pain or suffering, but it does remove hope. The concept of a virus as a deadly pathogen strikes fear into many people in a pandemic without recognising that of the most virus types on earth most are 'good' and vital to our existence, just as is the case with bacteria. God is not taken back by the coronavirus and even though it can be difficult to take on board he can work for the good even in the evil of it. When I recently asked the Bishop of Arundel and Brighton, Richard Moth, where is God in the pandemic, he replied that 'he is present in the sick and dying and in those who care for them', which can be of great help to those with faith. It is also important that the best medical advice is heeded, perspective is maintained, and love expressed. During pandemic, I personally enjoyed much greater contact with neighbours as we all tried to help each other while at the same time expressing thanks to doctors and healthcare workers. It was and is up to the individual to link this to a theist or atheist view. I was helped personally by the weekly 'Reflection' letter written during the pandemic by the Canon of Arundel Cathedral, David Parmiter, and many discussions with him. This gave me the opportunity to consider values at a time of crisis from his moral theological perspective and I chose to join the Catholic Church. Bioethics is a component of moral theology. Alongside all the natural, engineering, and social sciences, bioethical considerations are crucial as we determine the best means to preserve life on the planet.

7 The Path Ahead

INTRODUCTION

The future depends on what we do in the present.

Mahatma Gandhi 1869–1948

You can't connect the dots looking forward; you can only connect them looking backwards. So, you have to trust in something – your gut, destiny, life, karma, whatever. This approach has never let me down, and it has made all the difference in my life.

Steve Jobs 1955–2011

The pandemic clarified that science is inseparable from the rest of society and that connection works both ways. Science touches on everything; everything touches on science.

Ed Yong 1981–Present

Interdisciplinary conversations are extremely important on the huge matter of sustaining life. We need contributions from ethics, philosophy, politics, economics, and theology, as well as all the sciences. These conversations need to take place everywhere, including schools, universities, the media, government, and industry. I have tried to describe a picture of how life might have originated on this planet in cosmological terms, while also giving some ideas of how organisation of chemical molecules might have provided the framework for the origin of biological species from what was almost certainly a very small statistical chance. Inevitably much of what I have said in that respect is speculation and open to conjecture. It is important to continue to explore these concepts using a scientific approach which includes the use of engineering and social sciences.

We have seen during pandemic how sensitive we are to disease, but we should also recognise that all components of the biological universe are subject to an ever-present threat of pests and disease which can compromise humans by restricting food supplies. Even though climate has always been changing, the incontrovertible evidence is that we are entering a dangerous phase of warming to the planet. We have also become increasingly conscious that the planet itself and life on it will be compromised by climate change and that we need to use innovative scientific approaches as well as using political intervention, based on scientific evidence, to combat this problem. One major opportunity is to exploit the opportunities that mathematics presents for machine learning and artificial intelligence to quantify the problem and the potential solutions. Tipping point analyses will become increasingly important. The new powers of high-resolution satellite imagery for earth observation as a disruptive technology enables us to quantify how human action damages the planet; in

DOI: 10.1201/9781003304845-7

the same way, that increasingly powerful microscopic and imaging techniques allow us to quantify damage to our bodies. Consistent with what Mahatma Gandhi says all these actions today will govern our future life and longevity. It is important that such approaches are deployed in governance, such as setting a sensible price for carbon on the financial markets. This should include green bonds to give a long-term incentive for investors to be rewarded for protecting the environment, rather than allowing carbon-emitting industries merely to pay offsets for the damage they cause.

We need to generate initiatives from the most senior levels to promote the protection of the planet. It was mentioned in Chapter 3 that the Royal Family have been active in promoting environmental protection and at COP 26 the Queen in addressing world leaders said that we need to answer the call of reversing climate change for people of tomorrow, rise above politics and achieve true statesmanship. Using multiple approaches, we must cap global warming in 2100 to 1.5°C, but certainly a maximum of 2°C as agreed in the 2019 Paris COP 21, if we are to protect life on the planet and reach net zero emissions by mid-century. Unfortunately, at the last moment in Glasgow, India and China would not ratify the need to 'phase-out' coal power and would only agree to 'phase-down'. This meek outcome only just keeps the 1.5°C goal alive but it is not dead, and every effort must be made in the future in future meetings to protect nations that are particularly vulnerable to climate change. We must recognise that only around 11% of the world's total energy needs are currently met by renewable energy, and 78% of the total energy needs are met by oil, gas, and coal which cause runaway climate change. Pledges at COP 26, including the reduction of methane (80 times the warming power of carbon dioxide) emissions, might only reach an increase of 2.4°C, but so much will depend on action by countries after the Glasgow meeting. It will also involve massive social change to deliver the objectives. As a first step at the start of COP 26, even without the leaders of China and Russia, more than 100 world leaders signed a pledge to 'halt and reverse' deforestation globally by 2030. A total of £14 billion of public and private money will be focussed on the protection of Amazonia, Indonesia, and Congo. This certainly does not mean that we should reduce timber production, but rather more sustainable forestry practices, often avoiding clear-fell, with planned regeneration programmes. Hopefully, this will also be applied to the prevention of land degradation and generate more sustainable agriculture, which can include agroforestry. We should recognise that about 70% of the carbon stored on land is found in the soil, in part fed by the deposition from plant roots of about 40% of the carbon captured by plants as my work with John Whipps has shown. This is fed through rhizosphere microorganisms around roots as the drivers of the carbon budget and activity. This science is often ignored by those engaged in setting policy in this arena. Many of us have been making these arguments on carbon economies in land use and land use change for many years, but perhaps that now we are in 'last chance saloon' the ambition of halting global warming to be realised.

The Royal Society of Arts was founded in 1754 and in its early days, bearing in mind that around 3000 trees are needed to build a warship for the Navy, they persuaded the landed aristocracy to plant at least 60 million trees, not just for shipbuilding but for the beautification of the countryside. I was pleased to present a lecture on Trees for Life at their 350th anniversary in 2004, and that is ever more important the government fulfils its promises of extensive tree planting for a climate-change scenario. In the December 2021 issue of the *RSA Journal*, the strapline comment is that 'COP26 needs to be a turning point that precipitates the whole system we need to change'. Nicholas Stern, former chief economist at the World Bank author of *The Economics of Climate Change: The Stern Review* indicates that 'we need a new form of economic growth that breaks the destructive relationship between economic activity and the environment' and 'we have created the climate catastrophe, so resources in future will be far more valuable than if we had acted sensibly'. This is very much in line with the thinking of Tim Jackson discussed in Chapter 4. Also, in December the Foundation of Science and Technology held a meeting 'COP 26: Where do we go from here?' This was also a tribute to the Earl of Selborne who died during the year. There was consensus that we need to remain optimistic and continue to take advice of the Climate Change Committee, cut rhetoric on over-optimism of issues like hydrogen fuel, move to a more plant-based diet, and deliver on the Nationally Determined Contributions. We need nature-based solutions, particularly maintaining biodiversity, based on the outline produced by The Royal Society in October 2021 (Figure 7.1).

It was encouraging that Prince William launched in October 2021 *The Earthshot Prize: Repairing Our Planet*. He states that the modern world is at odds with the planet on which we live while trying to avoid being alarmist is in crisis. This will be tackled by providing five prizes each year of £1 million up to 2030 to generate change in the following arenas:

1. Protect and restore nature
2. Fix our climate
3. Clean our air
4. Revive our oceans
5. Build a waste-free world

These arenas are interactive. The award of the first five prizes was announced in October 2021. The first category was awarded to Costa Rica for their pioneering scheme which pays local people to restore natural ecosystems, reversing decades of deforestation and doubling the size of the country's forests. This has boosted ecotourism by $4 billion. We need more such initiatives at all levels. I recently visited the Jersey Zoo founded by Gerald Durrell where the whole focus is on wildlife conservation. It was great to see gorillas and orangutans in a beautiful parkland setting and making the public aware of the need to protect them globally. Jane Goodall launched her career in 1960 to protect chimpanzees in Tanzania and, as an environmental activist, is still spreading enduring hope at the age of 87 from her home in Bournemouth by video appearances. The seniority of such messages is good, but we also need young people to hear them and spread their own messages, a view also expressed by Barak Obama at COP 26.

Water is key to life, and in many parts of the world such as Africa, this is already limited. As glaciers melt, they initially move water. But as they shrink the supply dwindles and compromises agriculture in countries like Peru, along with the supply of fresh water to the capital Lima, generating a potential major crisis for which plans need to be made. Sustainable agriculture is key to our future, but we can learn so much from the past as well. For example, on my visits to Mexico, I have been impressed with the Chinampa agriculture system developed by the Aztecs (1345–1521) where small areas of fertile agricultural land on raised beds and crops are rotated were and still

Climate change impacts biodiversity through interactions with the Earth System.

Climate change induced factors such as earlier springs and changing ocean currents have consequences for all life on Earth. In turn, changes in biodiversity can impact the Earth System responses through changes to balanced cycles which further amplify climate change. Nature-based solutions (NbS) can help disrupt this cycle through the creation, restoration, management and protection of ecosystems to promote mitigation of and adaptation to climate change by altering the feedbacks between climate impacts and biodiversity, and Earth System responses. Examples of such NbS are outlined in the centre of the figure.

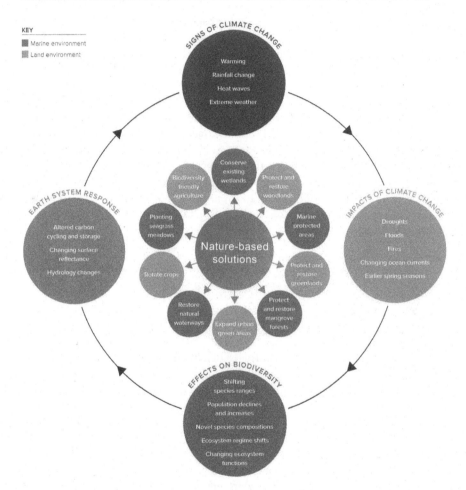

FIGURE 7.1 Climate change impacts biodiversity through interactions with the earth system. (From Climate change and biodiversity: Interlinkages and policy options, The Royal Society 2021. The text of this work is licensed under the terms of the Creative Commons Attribution Licence which permits unrestricted use, provided the original author and source are credited. The licence is available at: creativecommons.org/licenses/by/4.0 Issued: October 2021 DES7288 © The Royal Society.)

are effective in yield and free of pests and diseases. This is a long way from some of the modern high-intensity monoculture systems used today which are in my opinion unlikely to stand the test of time. The crofters of the West of Scotland and Ireland have harvested seaweed for centuries as an effective soil conditioner. Crab shells applied to the land have been used effectively in Kyushu, Japan, as an effective means of disease control in crops. Sustainability is not only key to global food security, but also to global health by minimising exposure to harmful chemicals.

Preventative health has been key in response to the pandemic, especially with the rapid development of vaccines which would not have been possible in the past without the in-depth analyses of DNA profile of the COVID-19 pathogen. Malaria, a disease caused by parasites following mosquito bites, is an even deadlier disease than COVID-19 in Africa where 386,000 people died compared with 212,000 coronavirus deaths in 2019. It was therefore great that the world's first malaria vaccine developed by the British pharma company GlaxoSmithKline, Mosquirix, was recommended for use in children by the World Health Organization in October 2021. Even though it has limited efficacy at present, preventing 39% of malaria cases and 30% of severe malaria cases in young children, it must surely only be a matter of time before a very effective vaccine is developed. The power to extend life will depend heavily on producing biochips which will be capable of diagnosing disease before even mild disease breaks out, unlike the current situation where early diagnosis is usually only possible at the boundary of moderate-severe disease and severe disease which leads to systemic failure. But the way, forward can also be relatively simple, aided by novel diagnostic technology, as well as new empirical science such as faecal transfer from healthy individuals to improve the health of the guts of people with problems, stimulating optimum microbiomes which will potentially improve the quality of life. Indeed, microbes will continue to play a major role in our future as they have in our origins and past.

An excellent example of novel diagnostics was reported in The Times on 16 April 2022 as I was correcting proofs for this book. My friend and colleague John Whipps referred to in this chapter and Chapter 5 was diagnosed with Parkinson's disease and 2007. He recently contributed to a study using smartwatches known as Parkinson's Kinetigraphs with Plymouth University, collecting information for 24 hours each day for six days as patients go about their daily lives, tracking sleep quality and any excessive movement or immobility, and buzz with reminders to take medication. Previously he was only assessed every six to 24 months by a consultant. In the same issue of the paper, it was reported that damaged hearts are being regenerated by scientists at King's College London using the same technology as coronavirus vaccines to develop a cure for heart attacks. The mRNA genetic codes that produce proteins that stimulate the creation of healthy heart cells have been identified and these could be potentially injected into heart attack patients by paramedics to prevent heart cells dying. We need to recognise that climate change will not only affect the crops we can grow to feed the world and the timber we can get from trees, but it also has the potential to set the fightback against human diseases. The *Lancet Countdown* on published in October 2021 on health and climate change was compiled by researchers from 38 academic institutions and UN agencies reviewed 44 indicators and points out the dangers of the delayed and inconsistent responses in the countries of the globe. It shows that climate change in threatening to reverse years of progress in public health and many healthcare systems are ill-prepared for climate-induced health shocks. To protect life, we need to combat the problem with clear international agreement. Artificial intelligence and machine learning techniques will be critical in this.

Steve Jobs unequivocally revolutionised the digital world and marketed the first personalised computer, providing a technology platform for the improvement of life. He was a self-proclaimed Buddhist, believing in higher consciousness, but not necessarily

God. Some have argued that his personality, especially in relation to the treatment of his family, is not to be admired. In the biography based on a series of interviews by and documented by Walter Isaacson *Steve Jobs* published in 2011, the year of his death, Jobs said 'Sometimes I believe in God, sometimes I don't. I think it's 50:50 maybe. But even since I've had cancer, I've been thinking about it a bit more. I kind of – maybe it's cause I want to believe in an afterlife. That when you die, it doesn't just all disappear. The wisdom you've accumulated. Somehow it lives on.' His wishes are consistent with the views of Stephen Hawking and Roger Penrose. For some, faith can provide the reality of those wishes and comfort to help to create a meaning to life. We have very big challenges now and, on the horizon, but we also have massive opportunities to capitalise on new science and technology. I fully support the views of Jane Goodall in her new book with Doug Abrams published in 2021 *The Book of Hope: A Survival Guide for an Engineered Planet*. Jane's four reasons for hope are:

- The Amazing Human Intellect
- The Resilience of Nature
- The Power of Young People
- The Indomitable Human Spirit

Without hope we are lost. She raises the issue that possibly life is a test and based on Bruce Greyson's research that near-death experiences transform how people live their lives and inspire a belief that there is a meaning and purpose in the universe. The inspirational beach sunset reflection picture in this book from my home in West Sussex (Figure 7.2) should not be seen as an ending, but for us to look forward to a bright sunrise. I support the Catholic view that there is no fundamental conflict between science and religion; science asks how things work and religion asks why there is any world at all. They are not mutually exclusive but interactive, and both are necessary to explain life and how it might be sustained. I for one am optimistic and have faith in God helping us to realise the new opportunities that science presents.

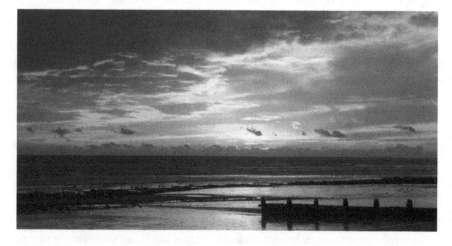

FIGURE 7.2   Reflections on a beach in West Sussex. (Photograph by Frans de Leij.)

Glossary

Agnostic	Existence of God is unknown or unknowable.
Anaerobe	Organisms capable of living in the absence of oxygen.
Anthropocentrism	Humankind is the central or most important of existence, as opposed to God or animals.
Archaea	Any group of prokaryotes that have distinct molecular characteristics which separate them from bacteria and eukaryotes.
Atheist	Compelling evidence against the existence of God.
Axiom	Like a postulate or assumption, it is a statement that is taken to be true and to serve as a premise or starting point for further reason and argument.
Big Bang	The dense hot beginning of the universe. The Big Bang theory postulates that about 13.7 billion years ago, the part of the universe we can see today was only a few millimetres across. Today, it is much larger and cooler, but we can observe remnants of the early period in the cosmic wave background radiation which permeates all space.
Biodiversity	A term that attempts to sum up the variety of life in the world. It is a function of the number of species, all different kinds of animals, plants and microorganisms, and the number, or abundance, that exists for each of those species.
Bioenergy	Renewable energy made from available materials in the natural world such as wood and sugar cane.
Bioethics	The ethics of biological and medical research.
Black hole	A region of space-time that, due to its immense gravitational force, is cut off from the rest of the universe.
BP	British oil company.
Carbon budget	The cumulative amount of carbon dioxide emissions estimated to limit global surface temperature to a certain level.
Carbon offset	A reduction in emission of greenhouse gases aimed to compensate for ongoing emissions elsewhere that cannot be afforded.
Carbon tax	A tax levied on the burning of carbon-based fuels aimed at getting the polluters to pay.
Chromosome	A thread-like structure of nucleic acids and proteins found in the nucleus of most living organisms, carrying genetic information in the form of genes.
CIA	Central Intelligence Agency in the USA.
Clear fell	Full removal of forest plantation.
COP	Conference of Parties – the UN Climate Change Conference

CRISPR	Clustered regularly interspaced short palindromic repeats – a segment of DNA containing repetitions of base sequences, involved in the defence of prokaryotic organisms to viruses.
Dark matter	This is a hypothetical form of matter thought to account for approximately 85% of the matter of the universe and about 27% of its total mass.
DDT	Dichlorodiphenyltrichloroethane insecticide.
Demiurge	A being responsible for the creation of the universe.
Determinism	The doctrine that all events, including human action, are ultimately determined by causes external to the will.
DNA	Deoxyribonucleic acid is a self-replicating material that is present in all living organisms as the main constituent of chromosomes.
Earth system	The integrated geological, chemical, physical, and biological system of planet Earth.
Ecological footprint	A measure of human impact on the environment.
Eukaryote	Organisms with complex cells, or single cells with complex structures, with genetic material organised into chromosomes in the cell nucleus.
Faith	Strong belief in the doctrine of religion, based on spiritual conviction rather than proof.
Forest dieback	The phenomenon of a stand of trees losing health and dying when a tipping point is reached.
Fullerenes	Molecules of carbon atoms with hollow shapes.
Genetic modification (GM)	Artificial alteration of the genetic material of an organism to produce a desired characteristic.
Greenhouse gases (GHG)	Gases that alter solar radiation and lead to the greenhouse effect which blanket the Earth to keep it at a higher ambient temperature.
Gross domestic product (GDP)	The value of goods and services provided in a year.
Heisenberg uncertainty principle	A law of quantum theory that certain pairs of physical properties cannot simultaneously to arbitrary precision.
Hominisation	Evolutionary development of human characteristics that differentiate hominids from their primate ancestors.
HRI	Horticulture Research International.
ICI	Imperial Chemical Industries (1926–2008).
Idealism	Unrealistic belief or pursuit of perfection.
Inundative release	The release of large numbers of mass-produced biological control agents or beneficial organisms with expectation of achieving a rapid effect.

Karma	The individual causal law which good or bad actions determine the future mode of an individual's existence (Indian philosophy and religion).
Metagenome	Genetic materials from environmental samples.
Metaphysics	The branch of philosophy that deals with the first principles of things, including abstract concepts such as being, knowing, identity, time, and space.
Microbiome	The combined genetic material of the microorganisms in a particular environment.
Moral theology	The branch of theology that deals with ethics, including bioethics. It is also termed Christian ethics, especially in the Anglican Faith.
M-theory	Prediction that a great many universes were created out of nothing, with many different possible histories. It is the unifying form of string theory.
Multiverse	Hypothetical group of multiple universes, which can also be called 'parallel', 'other' or 'alternative' universes or many worlds. They have space, time, matter, energy, and information.
Natural capital	Elements of the natural environment which provide valuable goods and services to people.
Natural regeneration	After felling a forest plantation, tree seeds are allowed to colonise the land and a stand of mixed trees, which can include deciduous and coniferous species, allowed to establish.
NDC	Nationally Determined Contributions to mitigate climate change, originally mooted at COP 21 in Paris.
Noosphere	A postulated sphere of evolutionary development dominated by consciousness, the mind, and interpersonal relationships.
OECD	Organisation for Economic Co-operation and Development.
Omega point	As humans interact consciousness evolves and grows, bound to the finite earth.
Palaeontology	The study of the history of life on Earth as based on fossils.
Parody	Imitation of the style of a writer with exaggeration, often to comic effect.
PCR	Polymerase chain reaction is a method to make millions of copies of a DNA sample to analyse it in more detail.
Prokaryote	Cellular organisms that lack an envelope-enclosed nucleus.
Quantum theory	A theory in which objects do not have single definite histories. It explains the nature of physics at the atomic and subatomic levels.
REDD+	A UN initiative Reducing Emissions from Deforestation and forest Degradation, and the role of conservation,

sustainable management of forests and enhancement of forest carbon stocks in developing countries.

Relativity theory   General relativity and special relativity are two interrelated theories of Albert Einstein. General relativity explains the law of gravitation and its relation to the other forces of nature, special relativity apples to all physical phenomena in the absence of gravity. For the latter, energy equals mass times the speed of light squared or $E = mc^2$.

Renewables   Energy from sources that naturally replenish themselves on a human timescale such as solar, wind, bioenergy, tidal, wave power, hydroelectric power, and geothermal heat.

Rhizosphere   The area of influence around plant roots.

RNA   Ribonucleic acid is a nucleic acid present in all cells, acting as a messenger (m-RNA) to carry instructions from DNA to control the synthesis of proteins.

Soil biotechnology   Study and manipulation of soil microorganisms and their metabolic processes to optimize crop productivity.

Space-time   Any mathematical model which fuses the three dimensions of space and one dimension of time into a single four-dimensional manifold. It can be detected in its individual quanta of matter and energy.

String theory   Theoretical framework in which point-like particles are replaced by one-dimensional objects called strings. The theory describes how the strings propagate through space and interact with each other.

Sudden oak death   Disease of oak trees caused by *Phytophthora ramorum*. Also called SOD

Sustainability   The ability for something to continue forever.

Tipping point   A threshold that, when exceeded, can lead to an abrupt, large, and often self-amplifying and potentially, irreversible change in the Earth system.

Top-down approach   The approach to cosmology in which the histories of the universe from top-down, that is, backwards from the present time.

Turing machine   Mathematical model of computation that defines an abstract machine that manipulates symbols on a strip tape according to rules.

UN   United Nations.

Uncertainty principle   Articulated by Werner Heisenberg in 1927 stated that the position and velocity of an object cannot be measured exactly at the same time, even in theory.

UNESCO   United Nations Educational, Scientific and Cultural Organisation.

Vitalism   Theory that the origin of life depends on a force or principle which is not just chemical or physical.

Bibliography

Al-Khalili, J. and McFadden, J. *Life on the Edge. The Coming Age of Quantum Biology.* 2014. Bantam Press.

Attenborough, D. *A Life on our Planet. My Witness Statement and a Vision for the Future. 2020.* Witness Books.

Baker, N. *The Strange Death of David Kelly.* 2007. Methuen Publishing.

Barrow, J. D. *Theories of Everything. The Quest for an Ultimate Explanation.* 1990. Oxford University Press.

Bramble, B. *Pandemic Ethics. 8 Big Questions of Covid-19.* 2020. Bartleby Books.

Breakwell, *G. Mistrust.* 2021. SAGE Publications.

Bruce, D. and Bruce, A. *Engineering Genesis. The Ethics of Genetic Engineering.* 1998. Earthscan.

Bryant, J.A. and La Velle, L. Introduction to Bioethics. 2019. Wiley Blackwell, Chichester

Calvin, M. *Chemical Evolution. Molecular Evolution toward the Origin of Living Systems on the Earth and Elsewhere.* 1969. Oxford University Press.

Carson, R. *Silent Spring.* 1962. Houghton Mifflin.

Chardin, P. T. de. *The Phenomenon of Man.* 1955. Editions du Seuil.

Christian, D. *Origin Story. A Big History of Everything.* 2018. Allen Lane.

Colwell, R. and Bertsch McGrayne, S. *A Lab of One's Own. One Woman's Personal Journey through Sexism and Science.* 2020. Simon & Schuster.

Davies, P.C.W. and Brown, J. eds. *Superstrings. A Theory of Everything.* 1988. Cambridge University Press.

Dawkins, R. *Outgrowing God. A Beginners Guide.* 2019. Bantam Press.

Dawkins, R. *The God Delusion.* 2006. Bantam Press.

Dixon, B. *Power Unseen. How Microbes Rule the World.* 1994. W.H. Freeman Spektrum.

Einstein, A. *The World as I See It.* 1935. John Lane: The Bodley Head.

Farrar, J and Ahuja, A. *Spike – The Virus v The People. The Inside Story.* 2021. Profile Books.

Fauci, A. *Fauci-Expect the Unexpected—Ten Lessons on Truth, Service, and the Way Forward.* 2022. National Geographic.

Francis, Pope. *Laudato Si'. On Care for Our Common Home. Encyclical Letter.* 2015. Our Sunday Visitor.

Freer-Smith, P. H., Broadmeadow, M. S. J. and Lynch, J. M. eds. *Forestry and Climate Change.* 2007. CABI.

Gates, B. *How to Avoid a Climate Disaster. The Solutions We Have and the Breakthroughs We Need.* 2021. Allen Lane.

Gleick, J. *Chaos. Making a New Science.* 1988. William Heinemann.

Goodall, J. and Abrams, D. *The Book of Hope—A Survival Guide for an Engineered Planet.* 2021. Viking.

Gore, A. *An Inconvenient Truth. The Planetary Emergency of Global Warming and What We Can Do About It.* 2006. Bloomsbury.

Gore, A. *Our Choice. A Plan to Solve the Climate Crisis.* 2009. Bloomsbury.

Goslett, M. *An Inconvenient Death. How the Establishment Covered Up the David Kelly Affair.* 2018. Zeus.

Hart, D. B. *The Experience of God. Being, Consciousness, Bliss.* 2013. Yale University Press.

Hawking, S. *A Brief History of Time. From the Big Bang to Black Holes.* 1988. Bantam Press.

Hawking, S. *Brief Answers to the Big Questions.* 2018. John Murray.

Hawking, S. and Mlodinow, L. *The Grand Design. New Answers to the Ultimate Questions of Life.* 2010. Bantam Press.

Hazen, R. M. *Genesis. The Scientific Quest for Life's Origin.* 2005. Joseph Henry Press.

Honigsbaum, M. *The Pandemic Century. A History of Global Contagion from the Spanish Flu to Covid-19.* 2020. WH Allen.

HRH Prince of Wales, Juniper, T. and Skelly, I. *Harmony. A New Way of Looking at Our World.* 2010. Blue Door.

HRH Prince Philip, Duke of Edinburgh. *Down to Earth.* 1988. William Collins.

Issacson, W. Steve Jobs. 2011. Simon & Shuster.

Jackson, T. *Prosperity without Growth. Economics for a Finite Planet.* 2009. Earthscan.

Kaku, M. *The God Equation. The Quest for a Theory of Everything.* 2021. Doubleday.

Lennox, J. C. *Where Is God in a Coronavirus World? 2020.* The Goodbook Company.

Love, J. and Bryant, J.A. eds. Biofuels and Bioenergy. 2017. Wiley Blackwell, Chichester

Lovelock, J. E. *Gaia. A New Look at Life on Earth.* 1979. Oxford University Press.

Lynch, J. M. *Soil Biotechnology. Microbiological Factors in Crop Productivity.* 1983. Blackwell Scientific.

Lynch, J. M. ed. *The Rhizosphere.* 1990. Wiley.

Lynch, J. M. and Hobbie, J. E. eds. *Microorganisms in Action—Concepts and Applications in Microbial Ecology.* 1988. Blackwell Scientific.

Lynch, J. M. and Poole, N. J. eds. *Microbial Ecology. A Conceptual Approach.* 1979. Blackwell Scientific.

MacKay, D. J. C. *Sustainable Energy – Without the Hot Air.* 2009. UIT.

Marshall, M. *The Genesis Quest. The Geniuses and Eccentrics on a Journey to Uncover the Origin of Life on Earth.* 2020. Weidenfeld and Nicolson.

McEvoy, J. G. *Leaving Christendom for Good. Church-World Dialogue in a Secular Age.* 2014. Levington Books.

McFadden, J. *Quantum Evolution. The New Science of Life.* 2000. Harper Collins.

Miller, J. *The Vaccine—Inside the Race to Conquer the COVID-19 Pandemic.* 2021. St. Martin's Press.

Morse, S. *Sustainability. A Biological Perspective.* 2010. Cambridge University Press.

Moseley, M. *Covid-19. What You Need to Know about the Coronavirus and the Race for the Vaccine.* 2020. Short Books.

Nurse, P. *What Is Life? Understand Biology in Five Steps.* 2021. David Fickling Books.

Penrose, R. *Shadows of the Mind. A Search for the Missing Science of Consciousness.* 1994. Oxford University Press.

Penrose, R. *The Emperor's New Mind—Concerning Computers, Minds and The Laws of Physics.* 1989. Oxford University Press.

Postgate, J. *Microbes, Music and Me. A Life in Science.* 2013. Mereo Books.

Ratzinger, J. and Bovone, A. *Donum Vitae. Congregation for the Doctrine of the Faith.* 1987. Catholic Truth Society.

Russell, B. *Why I Am Not a Christian.* 1957. Unwin Books.

Sagan, C. Cosmos. The Story of Cosmic Evolution. 1981. Macdonald & Co, London

Scola, A. *Gaudium et Spes. On the Church in the Modern World.* 1966. Catholic Truth Society.

Tree, I. *Wilding. The Return of Nature to a British Farm.* 2018. Picador.

Vince, G. *Adventures in the Anthropocene. A Journey to the Heart of the Planet We Made.* 2014. Chatto & Windus.

Waksman. S.A. *My Life with Microbes.* 1958. The Scientific Book Club.

Index

Note: *Italic* page numbers refer to figures.

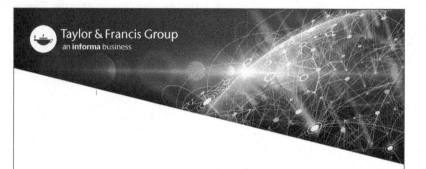